The Funny Side Collection

The Fart Side

Bottoms Up!

(Pocket Rocket Edition!)

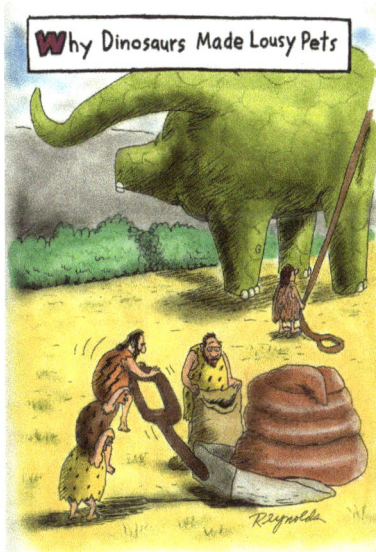

Dan Reynolds

Joseph Weiss, MD

© 2017 Dan Reynolds
　　　Joseph Weiss, M.D.
　　　SmartAsk Books
　　　Rancho Santa Fe, California, USA
　　　www.smartaskbooks.com

ISBN-13: 978-1-943760-50-3 (Color Pocket Rocket)
ISBN-13: 978-1-943760-51-0 (e-Book Pocket Rocket)
ISBN-13: 978-1-943760-57-2 (Color Print Expanded)
ISBN-13: 978-1-943760-62-6 (e-Book Expanded)

The Fart Side: Bottoms Up!

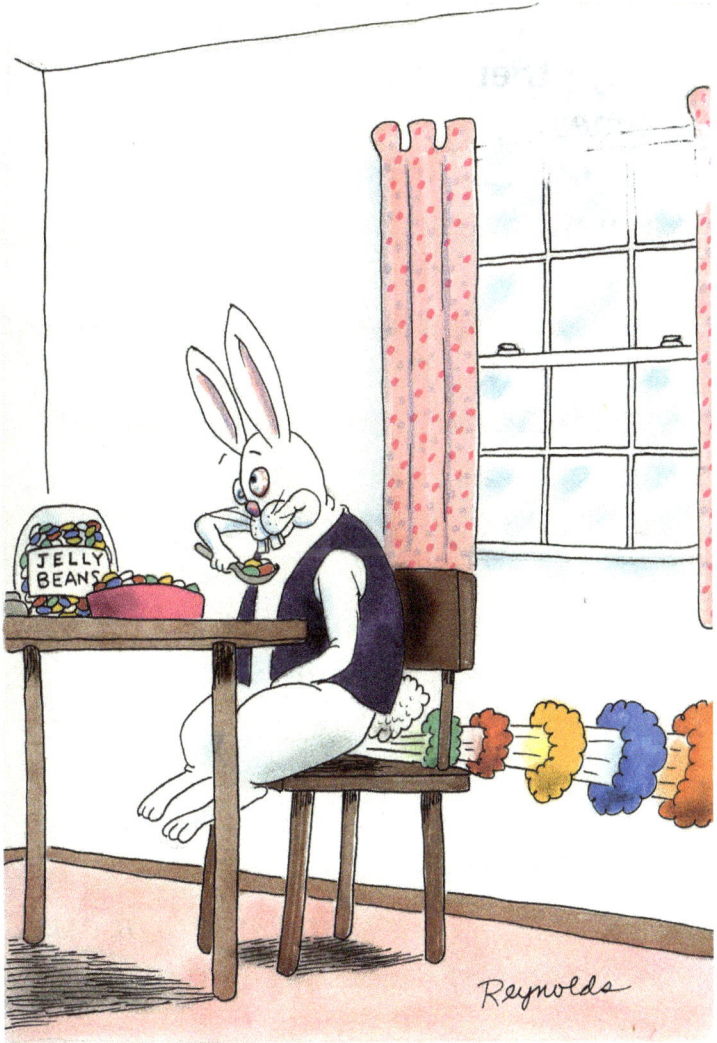

Methane is not produced by bacteria, but by other microbes known as Archaea.

The flammability of intestinal gas results when methane and/or hydrogen are produced. If the ignited gas has a blue flame it signifies that methane is present. The lighting of intestinal gas is not without risk and can lead to injury.

If the average person parts 14 times a day, by 80 years of age they will have farted about 41,000 times.

Because humans continue to regress even as technology progresses, there are at least 60 apps for smart phones which recreate the sound of human flatulence.

The Fart Side: Bottoms Up!

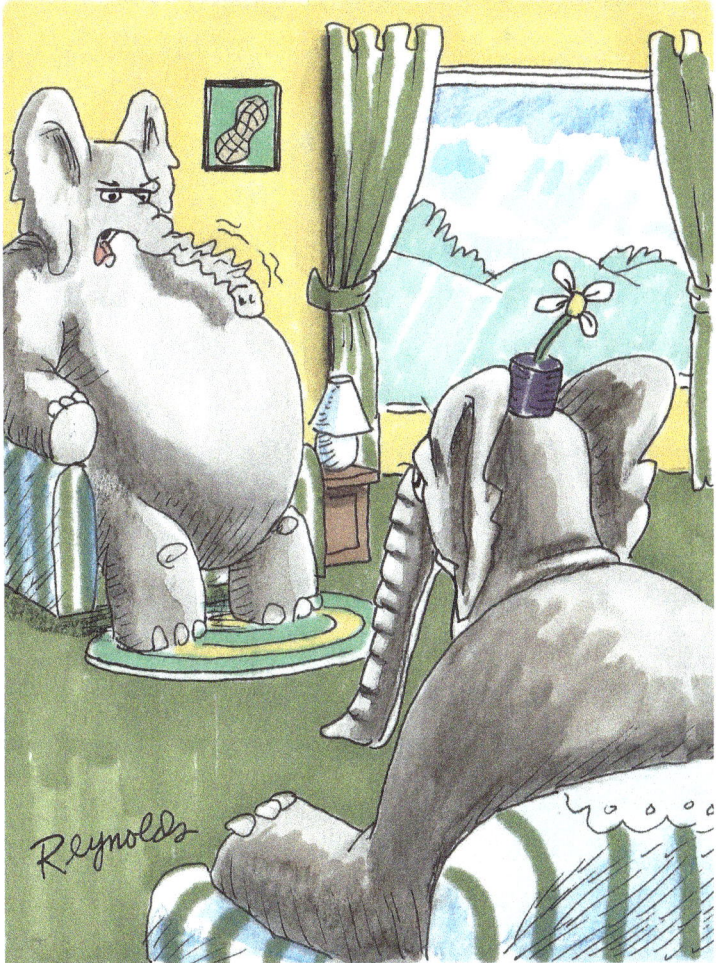

The Ontario Ministry of Health embarked on a public education campaign to curb tobacco usage. A common theme used by smokers to avoid the stigma of nicotine addiction was to describe their habit as a social smoker. The public education campaign focused on the denial as being analogous to describing oneself as a social farter, that is a person who enjoyed farting while in the company of others.

Pythagoras of Samos (c.570 BCE - c.495 BCE) was a Greek philosopher and mathematician from the region of Ionia. Pythagoras demanded that his adherents and students abstain from eating beans to avoid flatulence, as he believed that with every fart a small portion of the soul escaped.

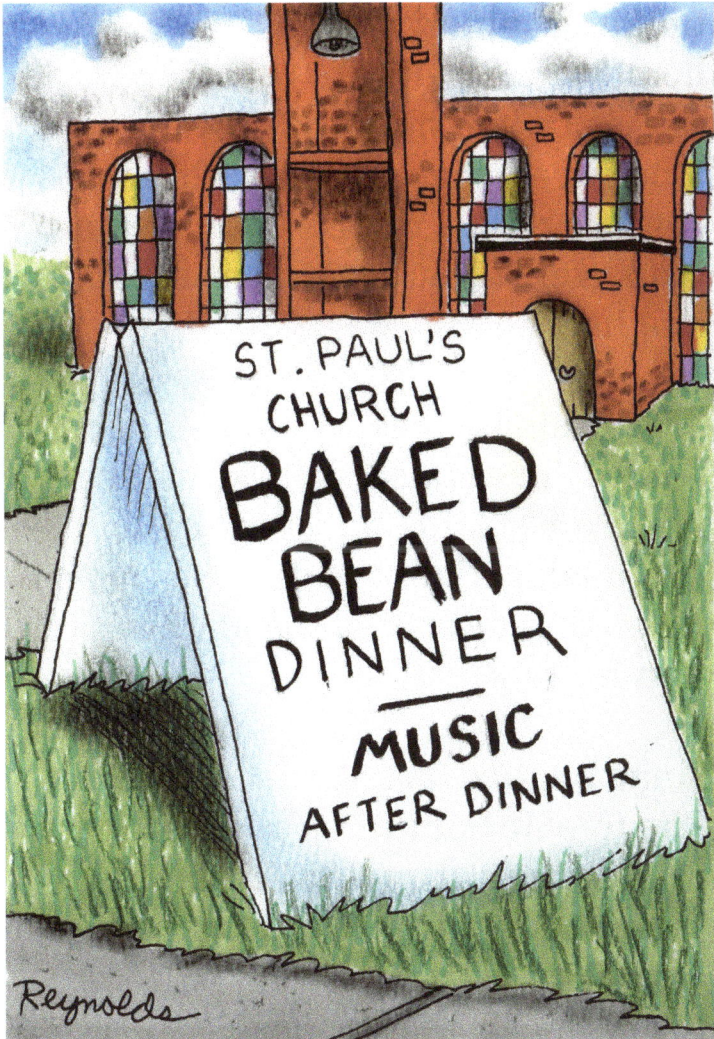

Inhaling some farts may be healthy. According to researchers at Exeter University, sniffing tiny amounts of hydrogen sulfide can reverse mitochondrial damage and help avert strokes, dementia, cancer, and heart attacks.

"Professional Fart Smeller" is a job in China. These talented professionals make up to $50,000 a year by diagnosing digestive illnesses merely through the scent of the patient's flatulence.

Some beetles fart to attract mates. The female Southern Pine Beetle releases sex attractant hormones, known as pheromone, in their farts to attract male suitors.

The Fart Side: Bottoms Up!

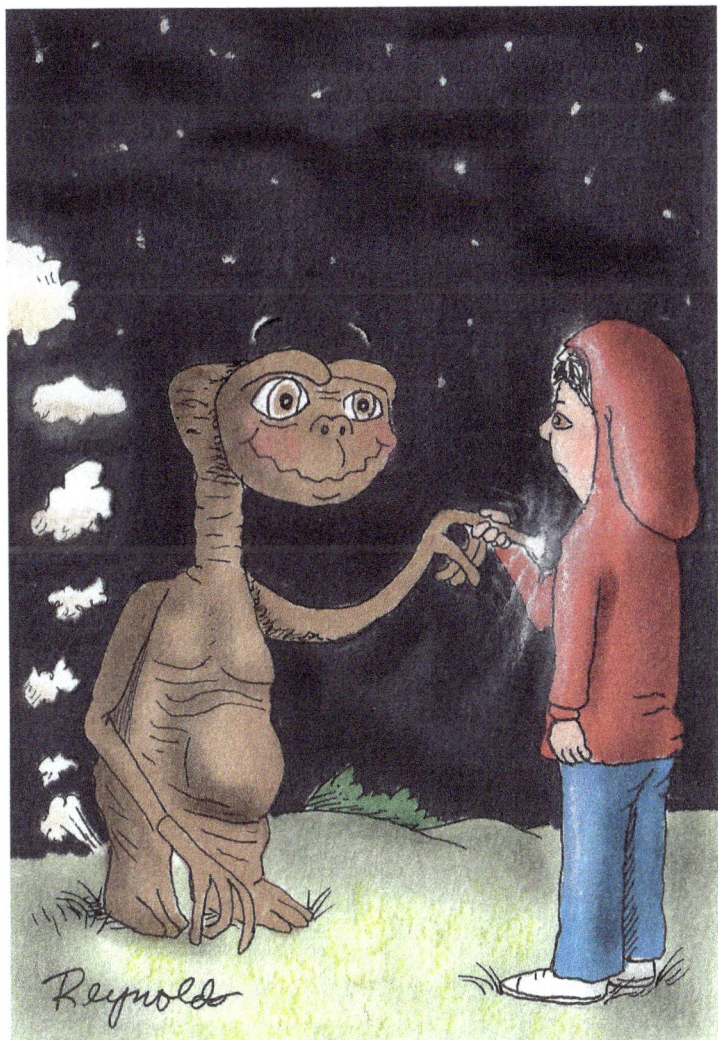

There is a marine creature that farts into its own mouth. Crinoid, also known as the "Sea Lily", has an intestinal tract that is U-shaped, which means that its flatulence is released right near its own mouth.

Half of all women admit that they have farted during sex. According to a study at the University of California San Francisco-East Bay, 43% of women surveyed reported that they'd experienced 'flatus incontinence' with sex over the previous three months. Males refused to admit that they had a similar release as well.

Elagabalus, a Roman Emperor who was assassinated at age eighteen, was known for using whoopee cushions as a practical joke.

The Fart Side: Bottoms Up!

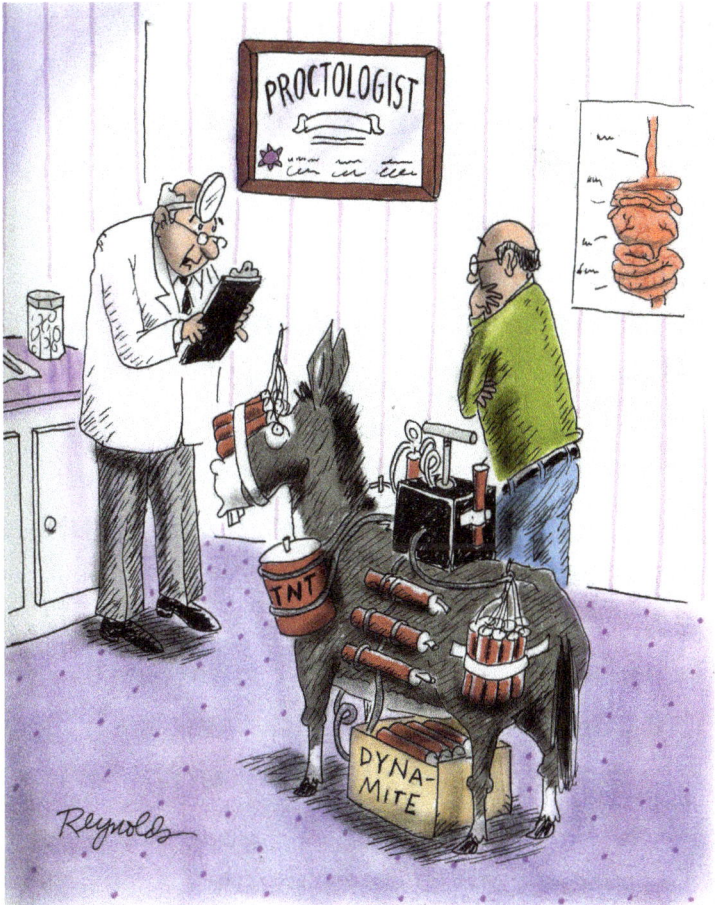

"Mr. McCarthy, you have a condition known as Explosive Ass Syndrome."

According to tradition, Germans considered it highly impolite if their guests did not burp. It's a way of telling the host that you are satisfied.

German priest and religious reformer Martin Luther used to say, *"Warum pfurzet und ruelpset ihr nicht, hat es euch nicht geschmecket?"* which translates to, *"Why don't you farteth and burpeth? Didn't you fancy the meal?"*

Women release greater quantities of the gas hydrogen sulfide, which has a foul rotten egg smell, in their farts than men.

The name mammal is derived from mammary glands, the medical term for the breasts which produce milk.

The Fart Side: Bottoms Up!

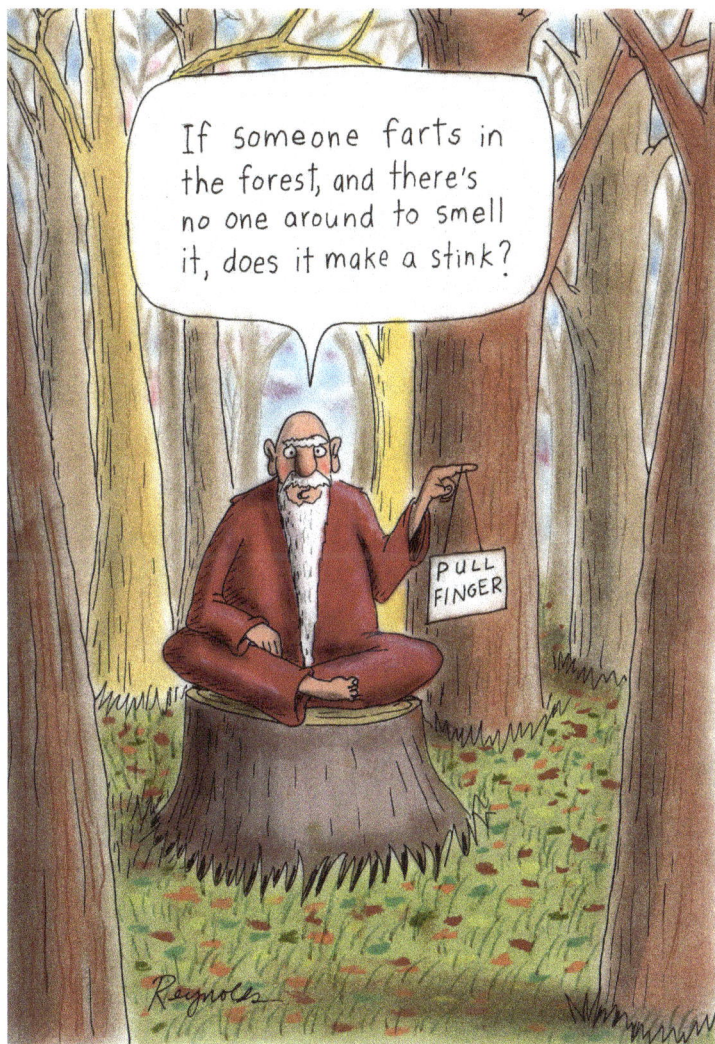

Aristotle (384 BC – 322 BCE) was a prominent Greek philosopher and polymath. He was a student of Plato, and the teacher and friend of Alexander the Great. Aristotle wrote on the digestive problems of elephants in his work *Historia Animalium*. He correctly described Elephants as having flatulence.

Nearly thirty thousand trees a day are converted into toilet paper.

Cicero's famous Farticus was possibly the world's first limerick:
There once was a man named Farticus
Who bravely fought beside Spartacus.
He let one rip,
His gladius slipped,
And we smelled no more of this Farticus.

The Fart Side: Bottoms Up!

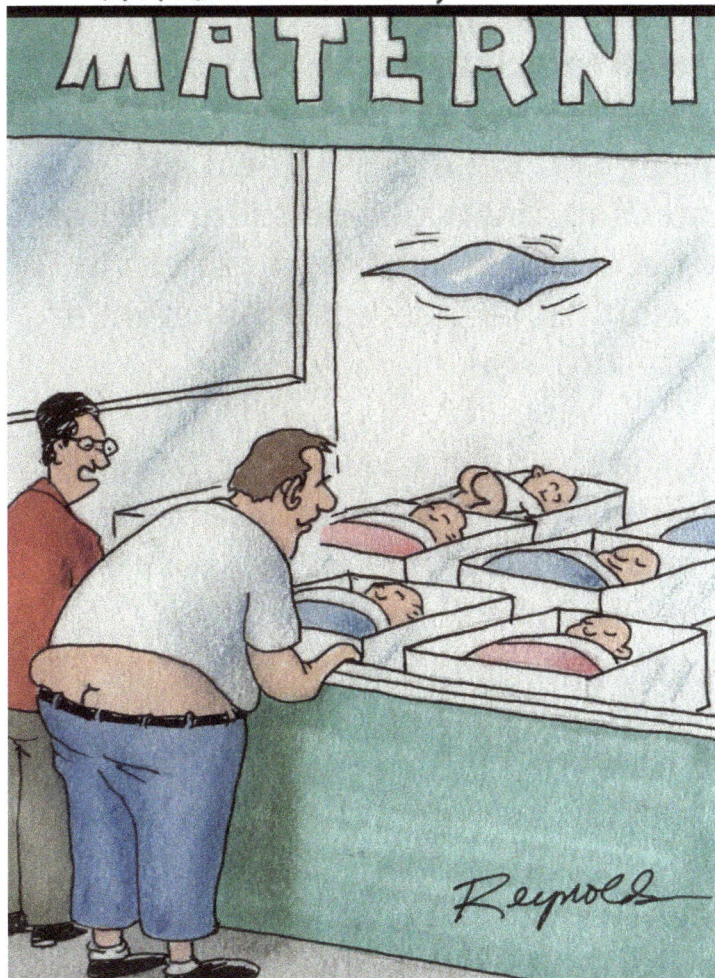

"Which one is yours?"

Even though they are dairy products, hard cheeses and yogurt often have relatively low lactose content.

A high fat meal slows down gut motility and transport, allowing more microbial fermentation, which results in the greater production of intestinal gas.

Although most farts are invisible under ordinary circumstances, it is not difficult to make them readily visible by farting underwater.

Hydrogen sulfide is a poisonous gas with a rotten egg smell that the human nose can detect at very low concentrations. When the gas concentration is high, the nose cannot detect it at all.

The Fart Side: Bottoms Up!

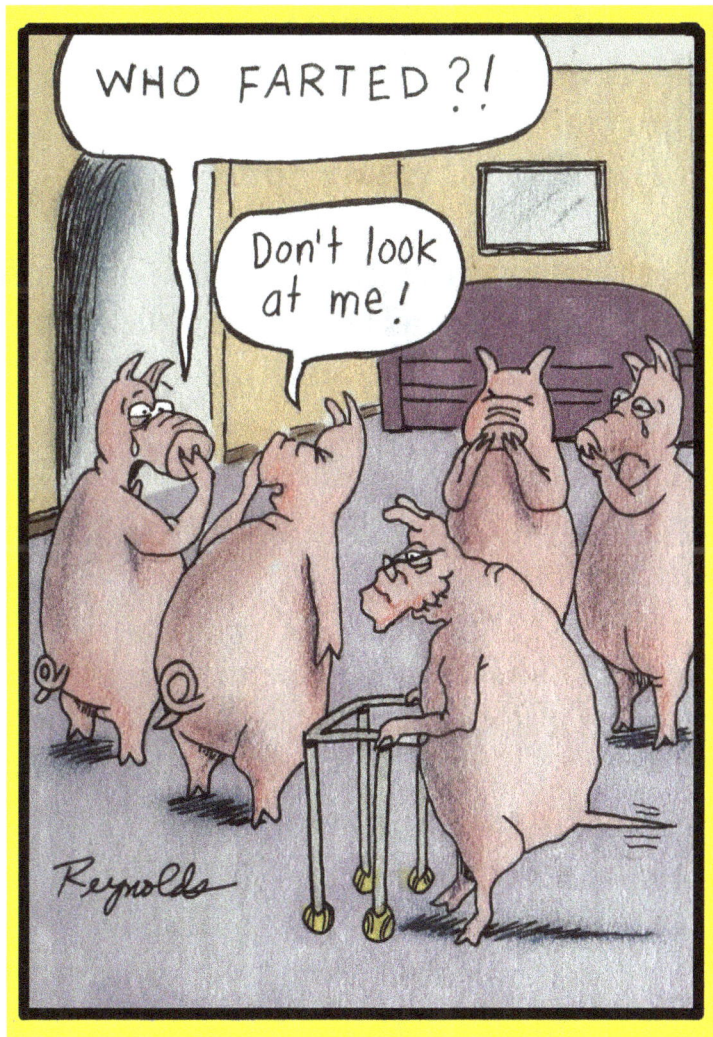

Farting is more likely to occur in elevators while they are going up in high rise buildings than in those exact same elevators going down.

The potency and aroma of the farts of boys increases as they go through puberty and reach adulthood.

Females have a heightened sense of smell at the time of ovulation during the menstrual cycle.

William Shakespeare refers to a fart in one of his plays.

US President Lyndon Johnson insulted future US President Gerald Ford by claiming he wasn't smart enough to be able to chew gum and fart at the same time.

Her toes in the sand. The wind at his back. They were living the dream.

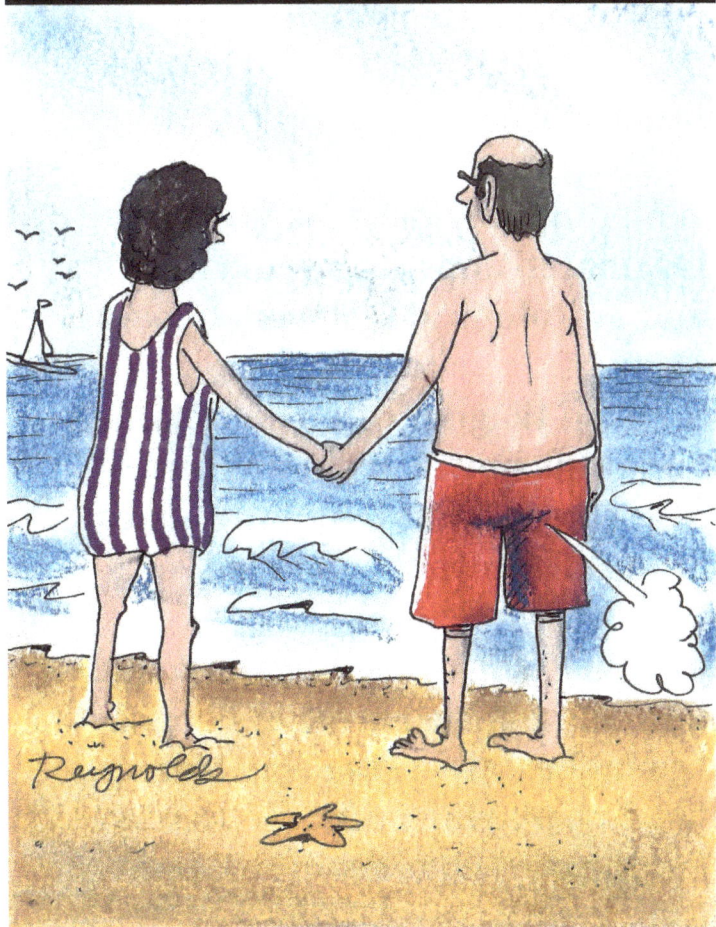

The Funny Side Collection

Roman Emperor Claudius decreed that citizens of Rome could fart in public, because he believed that holding back a fart could lead to illness or death.

Wolfgang Amadeus Mozart was fascinated and obsessed with farts and scatological matter.

Richard Wagner often complained about his bowel problems and described his farts by the musical notes and keys they played.

Joseph Pujol, known by the name Le Pétomane (The Farter in French) was the highest paid stage performer of his day, playing Le Marseilles by farting out the tune on the Moulin Rouge in Paris.

The Fart Side: Bottoms Up!

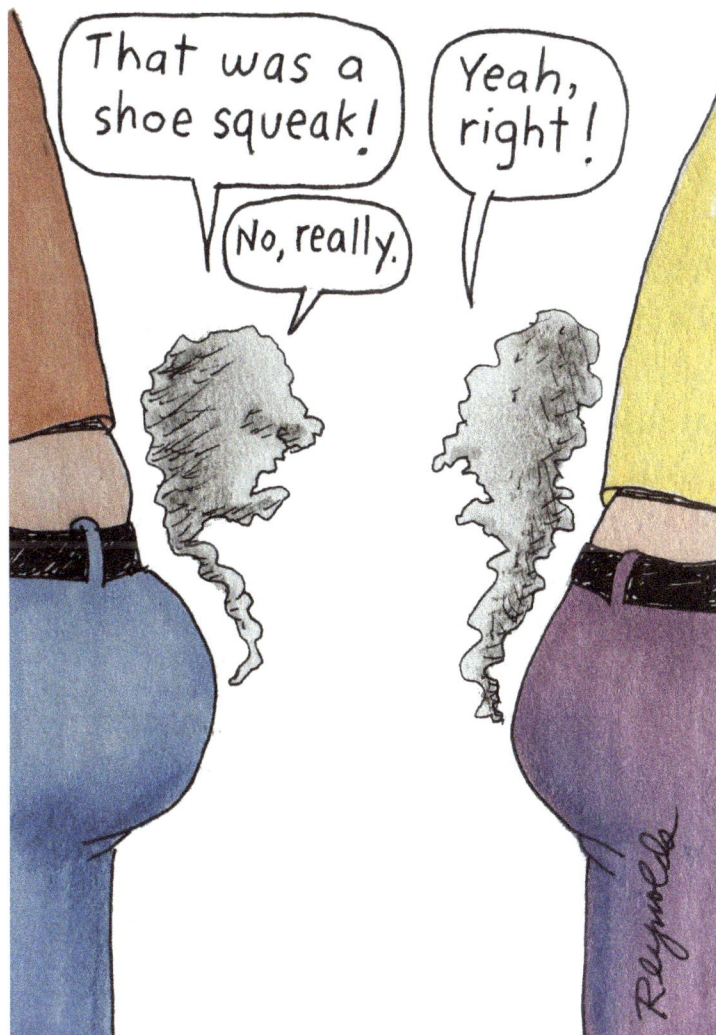

Prominent fart scenes have occurred in hundreds of Hollywood movies, including Walt Disney films for children.

The famous Greek mathematician Pythagoras believed that beans should not be consumed because a small portion of the soul escaped with each fart. He was so opposed to harming bean plants that he refused to flee across a bean field to escape from the assassins who killed him.

Over four billion people around the world never use toilet paper.

The average speed of a fart is indirectly measured by the diffusion of its smell, which has been recorded as greater than ten miles per hour.

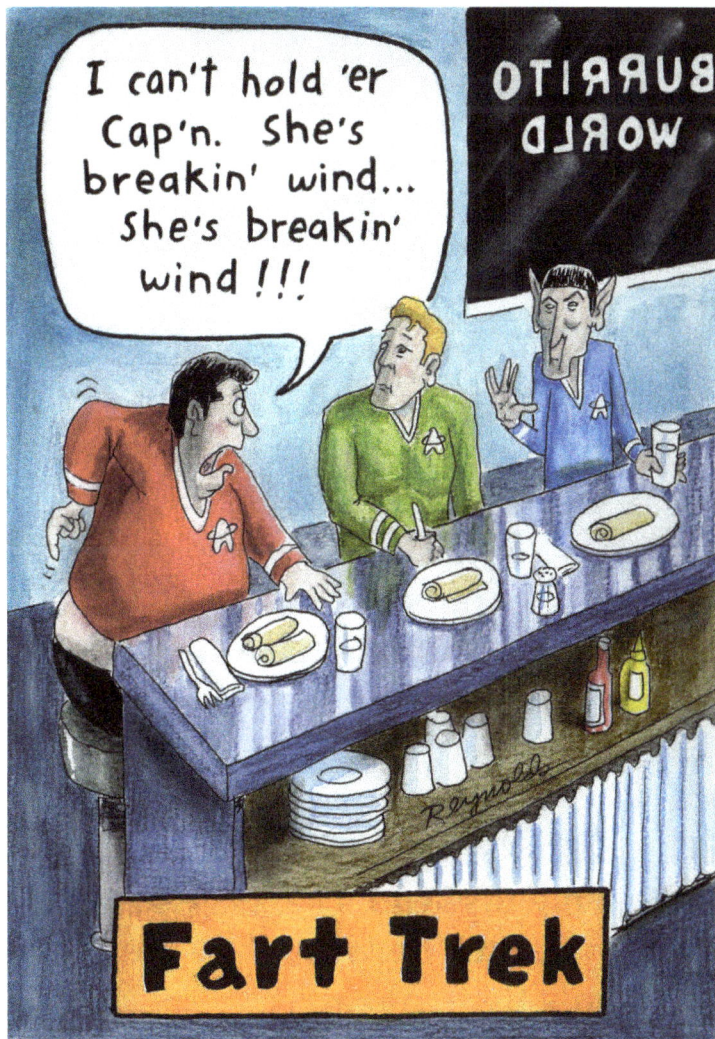

Morticians secure the anus of the deceased closed so that an audible fart from the corpse or casket does not frighten attendees at a memorial service or funeral.

Farting has become more accepted in Western society, with frequent references to it and the treatments available, in the media.

Using toilet paper is not hygienic, as the paper is thin and porous. Toilet paper is an inferior form of cleansing compared to water from a bidet.

The pastry delicacy Pets de Nonne, which means 'Nun's Farts' in French, is named such because they are heavenly light and airy.

The Fart Side: Bottoms Up!

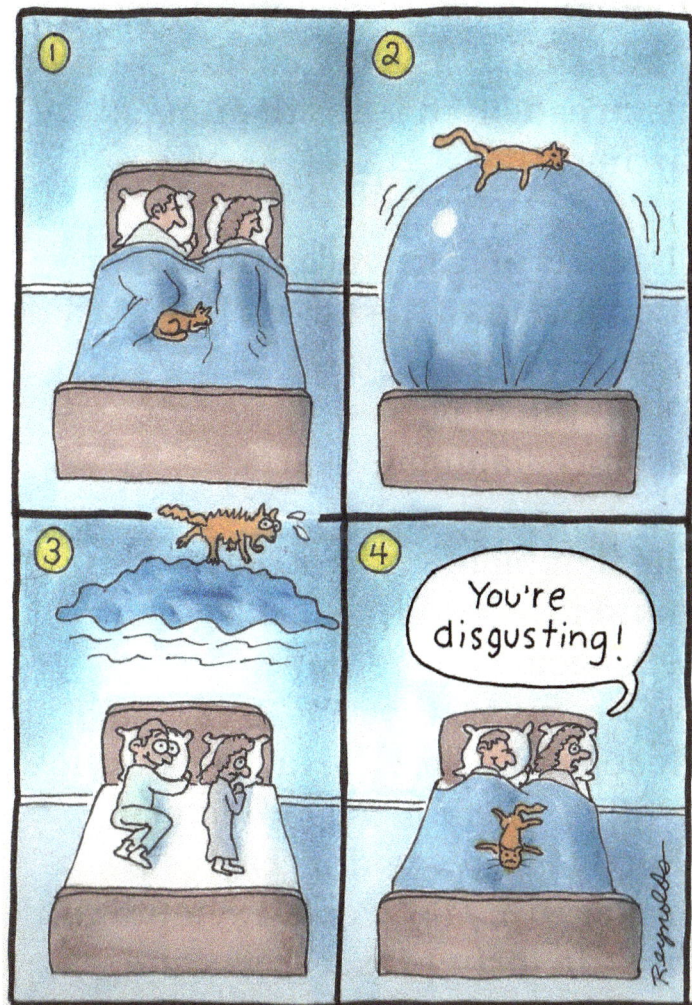

Pumpernickel is the German word for 'Devil's Farts and the coarse grain of the bread often leads to pungent farting.

The farts of carnivores smell more offensive than the farts of vegetarians

About thirty percent of people produce flammable farts.

The flammable gasses that may be found in a fart include oxygen, hydrogen, and methane.

Most people lose the lactase enzyme to digest the milk sugar lactose shortly after weaning. Lactose intolerance may exhibit symptoms that can include excess gas and cramps.

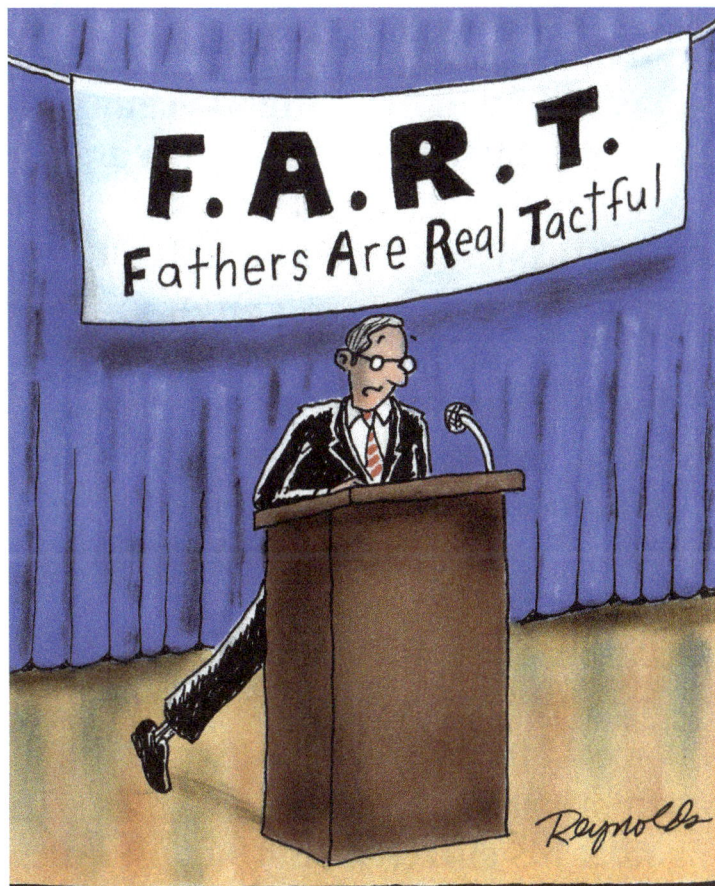

Despite their efforts to be credible, the pro-dad group did nothing but raise a stink.

Metrocles (c.325 BCE), a philosopher who studied in Aristotle's Lyceum, accidentally farted in public while practicing a speech. He was so embarrassed that he attempted to commit suicide by starvation.

Tiberius Claudius Caesar Augustus Germanicus (13 BCE – 54 AD), commonly known as Claudius, became the fourth emperor of the Roman Empire upon the assassination of his predecessor Caligula. Claudius had been made aware of an individual who had died as the result of a retained fart. To protect his citizens from a similar ill wind of fate, he decreed that all citizens of Rome could fart at will in public or in private.

Mom, Dad said he was bitten by a radioactive stink bug which gave him a superpower. What is it?

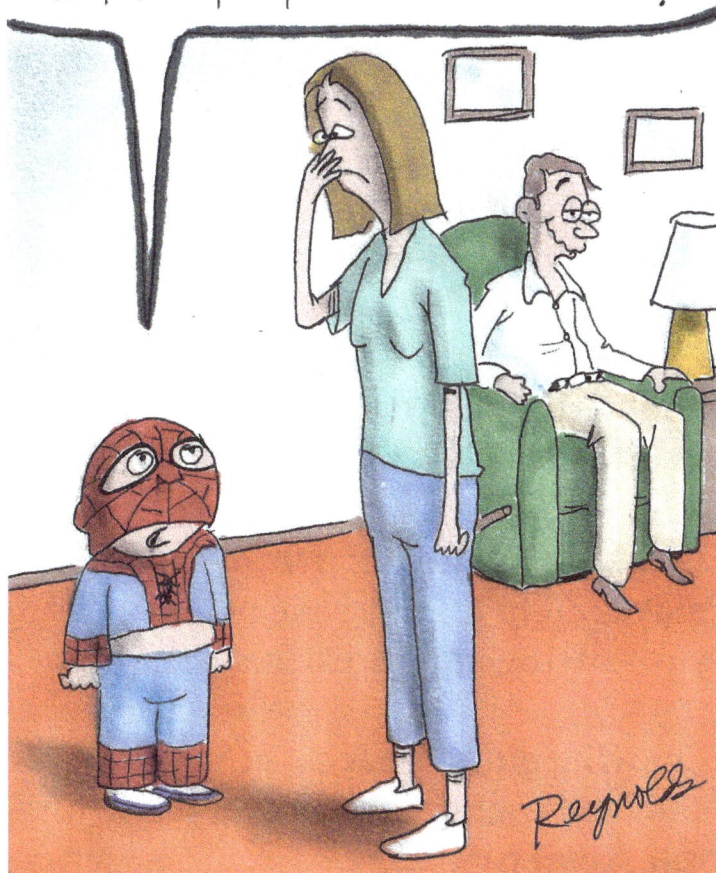

An apple is forty percent air by volume, and contributes to intestinal gas.

Meteorism is an old English term for farting.

Women and girls fart with the same frequency as men, but in smaller volumes.

Poor fitting dentures can contribute to intestinal gas by air swallowing.

Drinking from a straw, bottle, or can may lead to an increase in air swallowing and intestinal gas.

Chewing gum, tobacco, or ruminating can lead to increased aerophagia and intestinal gas.

The Fart Side: Bottoms Up!

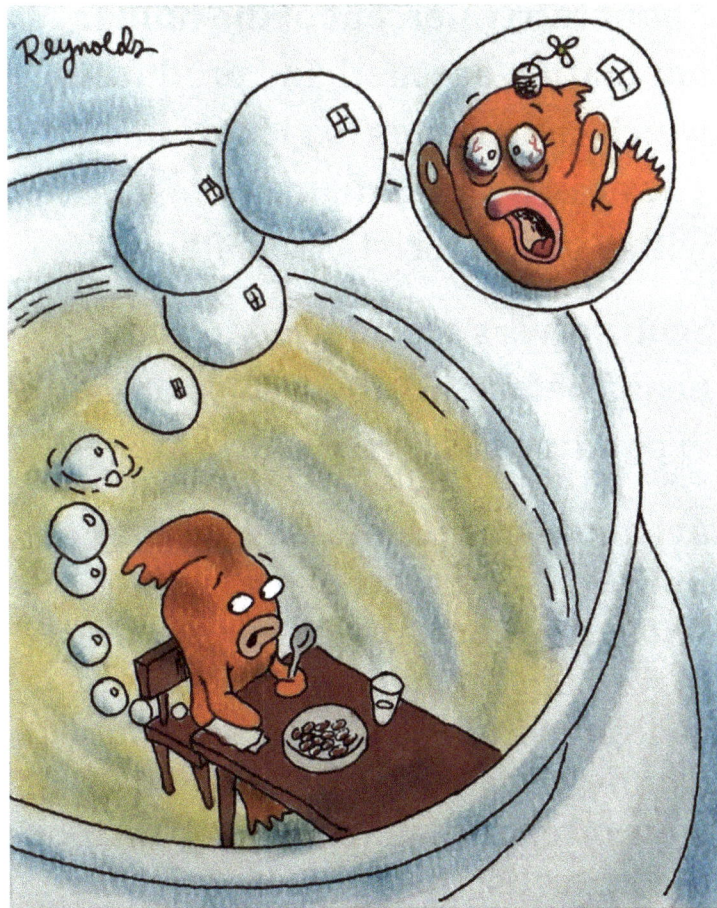

"Your baked beans are out of this world, honey... honey???"

About thirty percent of the human population are methane producers, which contributes to global warming. They can produce flammable farts with a characteristic blue flame.

Scuba divers are advised to avoid beans before a dive because of the expanding gas issue on ascent.

Aristophanes (c. 446 BCE – c. 386 BCE) was a comical playwright of Ancient Greece. His 5th century BC plays The Knights and The Clouds, contain numerous fart jokes. *The Clouds*:" First, think of a tiny fart that your intestines make. Then consider the heavens: their infinite farting is thunder. For thunder and farting are, in principle, one and the same.

The Fart Side: Bottoms Up!

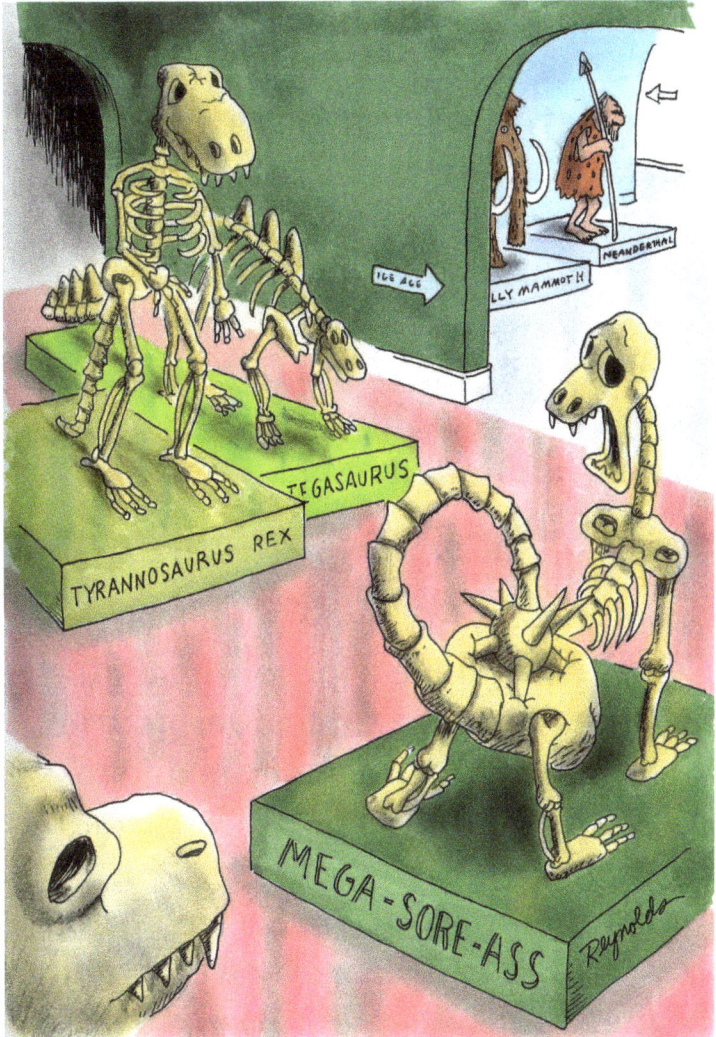

The ten liters of air swallowed every day by the average person is seventy-eight percent nitrogen. Nitrogen is not well absorbed by the intestinal tract and must be released as either a burp or as a fart.

Most people burp and fart while they sleep, and occasionally it is loud or aromatic enough to wake themselves or a sleeping partner.

Beer poured in the mile-high city of Denver will have a larger head of bubbles than the same beer poured in Seattle. The difference is due to atmospheric pressure and altitude.

Gelato compared to ice cream has a lower calorie content by weight, but a higher calorie content by volume.

The Fart Side: Bottoms Up!

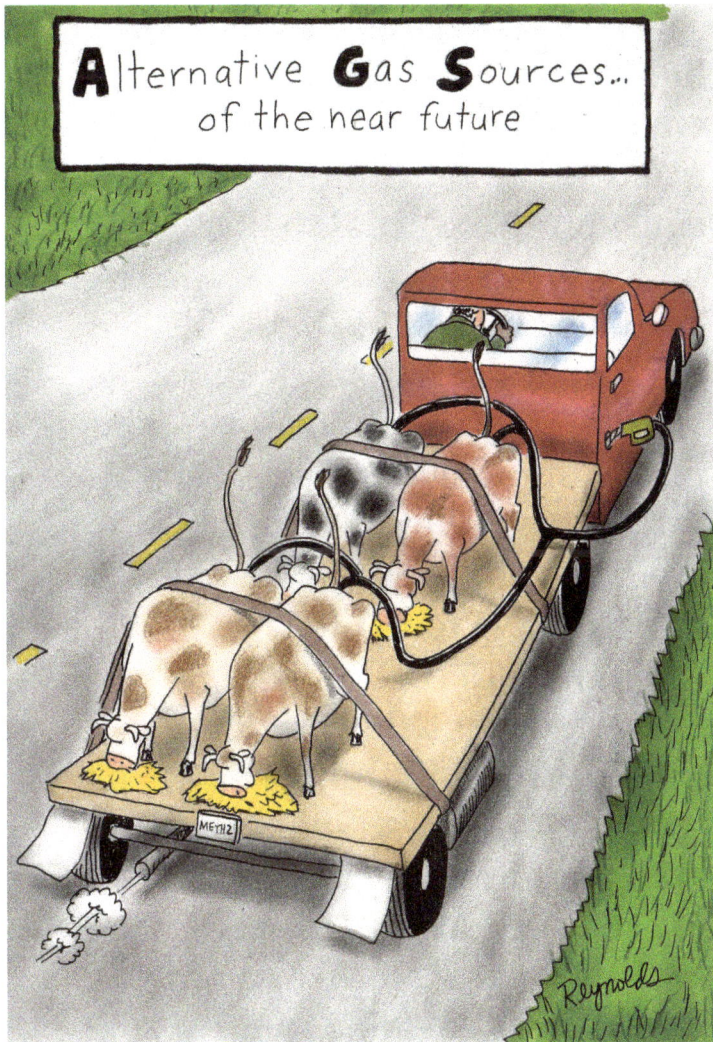

Alternative **G**as **S**ources...
of the near future

The largest organ or tissue of the body exposed to the external environment is the gastrointestinal tract. The inside lumen of the gut is considered external to the body.

Thomas Moore (1478 – 1535) was a philosopher, statesmen, humanist, and theologian, who was canonized to sainthood by the Pope. King Henry VIII beheaded him when he refused to accept papal authority regarding his marriage to Catherine of Aragon. In 1518, Sir Thomas More, in an epigram entitled *In Efflatum Ventis*, wrote "'Wind, if you keep it too long in your stomach, kills you; on the other hand, it can save your life if it is properly let out. If wind can save or destroy you, then is it not as powerful as dreaded kings?'"

The Fart Side: Bottoms Up!

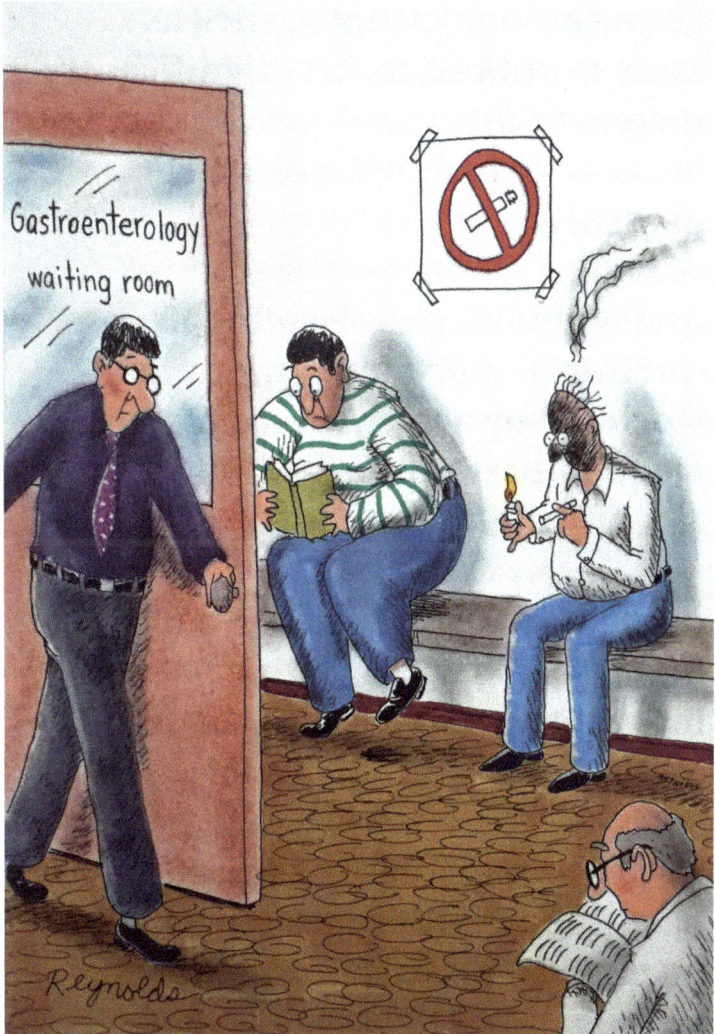

Living at high altitude, such as Denver or Mexico City, significantly increases intestinal gas volume because of lower atmospheric pressure.

Anal scent glands are often used as territorial markers in the animal world. They are one reason dogs are frequently smell each other's butts to identify their scent.

Going up in an elevator in a high-rise building increases farting because intestinal gasses expand as the atmospheric pressure decreases.

The US Department of Agriculture has supported research to develop a bean with lower concentrations of the sugars that lead to flatulence.

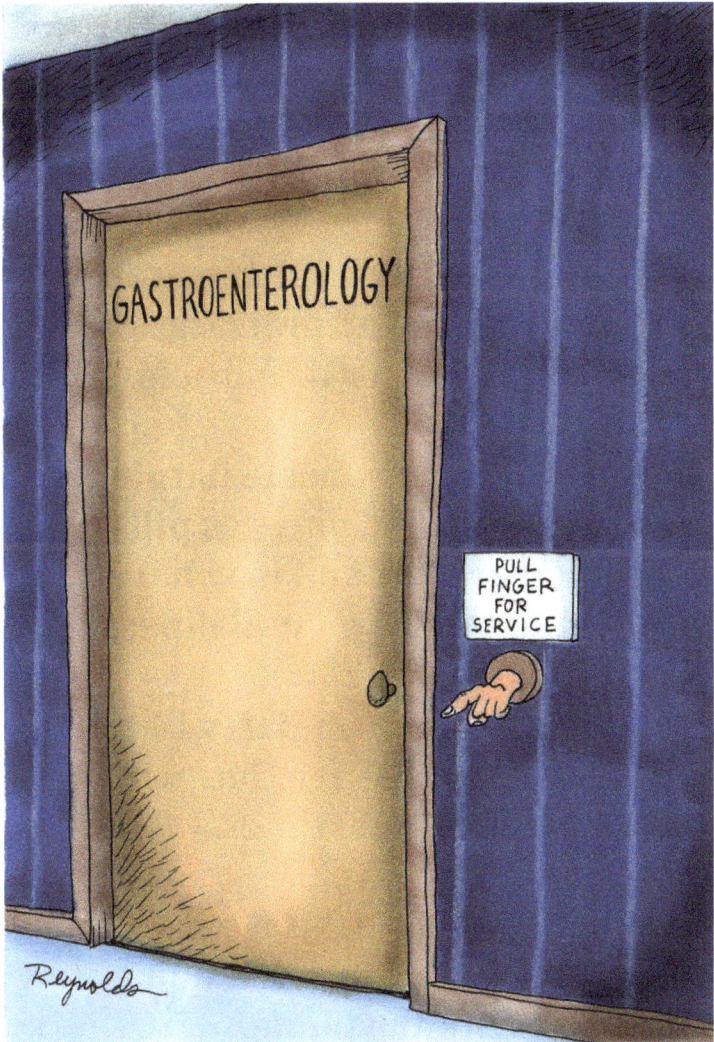

Although about thirty percent of people enjoy the aroma of their own farts, a smaller percentage enjoys the aroma of the farts of others.

The psychiatric condition of deriving sexual pleasure and gratification from farts is known as eproctophilia.

Adolf Hitler had extreme flatulence. He was prescribed anti-gas pills that contained arsenic and may have contributed to his mental illness.

If the average person parts 14 times a day, by 80 years of age they will have farted about 41,000 times.

Burping after a meal is a compliment to the hostess in several Asian cultures including China.

The Fart Side: Bottoms Up!

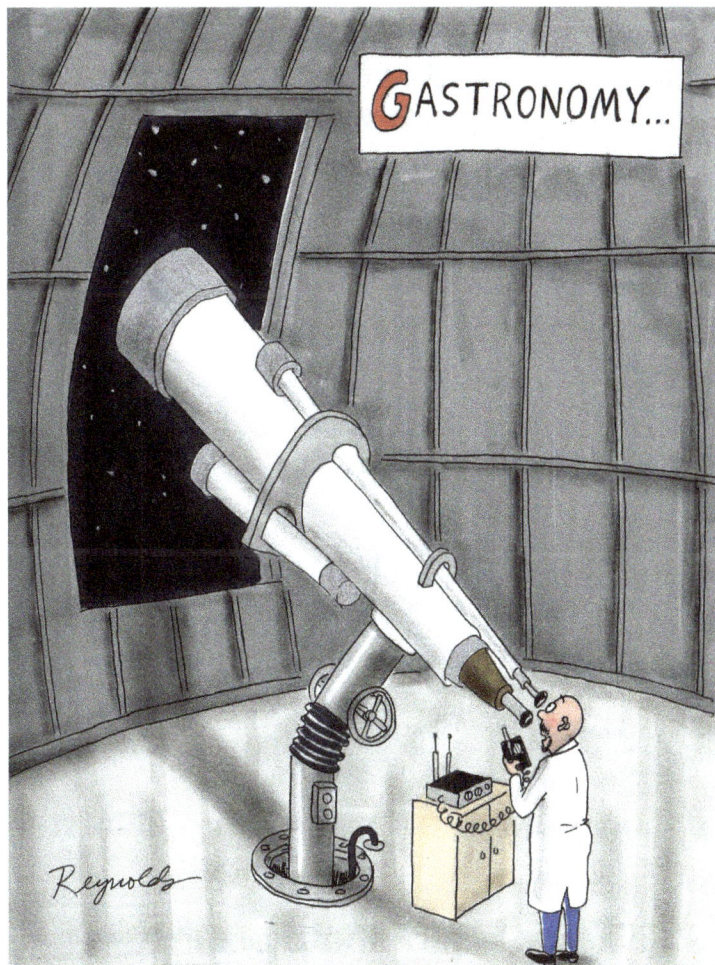

"I can't see a thing. The poisonous gases are covering Uranus."

How fast does a fart travel? About 10 feet per second, which works out to about 7 miles per hour. At that rate, it would take a fart a little more than three hours to run a standard marathon.

The average speed of a fart leaving the anus is about 10 feet per second or about 9.5 km/hr.

Gerald Ford, 38th U.S. President would blame his farts on the Secret Service by loudly proclaiming "Jesus, was that you? Show some class!"

Carbon Dioxide gas is easily absorbed by the gut, enters into solution in the blood, and is eliminated from the body by being exhaled via the lungs.

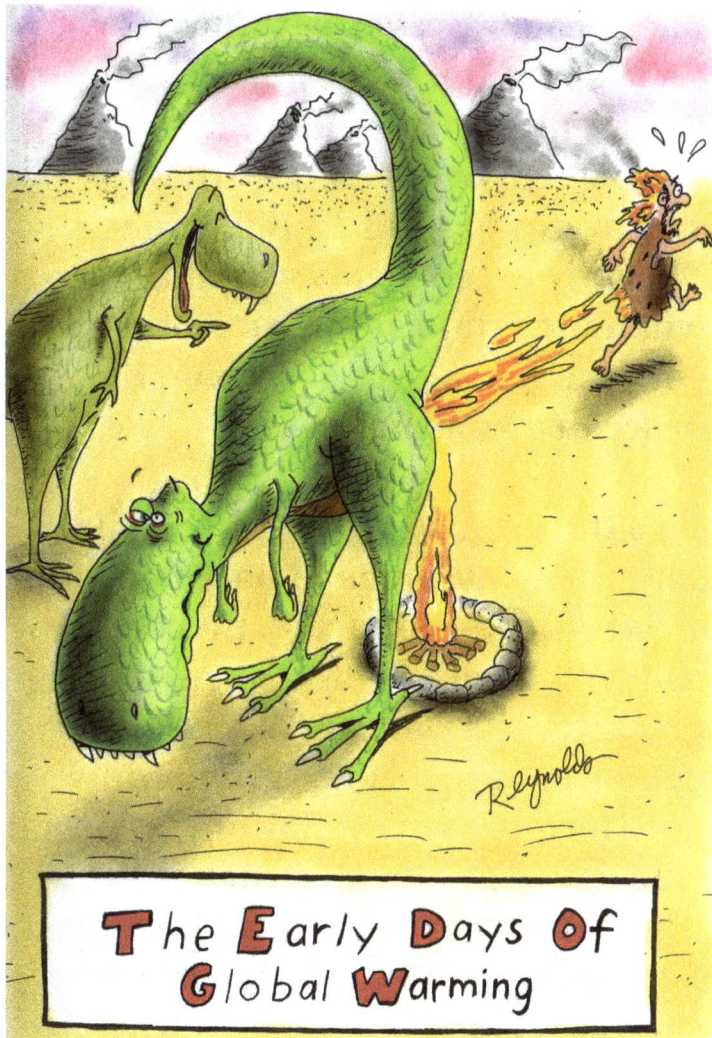

The Early Days Of Global Warming

The sensory nerves within your rectum can tell the difference between a fart and poop. They can distinguish between the different sensations of solid, liquid, and gas. The only exception is with diarrhea when the liquid stool can be released with the passage of gas, commonly described as a shart.

Two thirds of adults pass farts that contain no methane. If both parents are methane producers, their children have a 95% chance of being producers as well. Since methane producers are an elite group (only one third of the population), a special club called the Royal Order of the Blue Flame has been established just for that them. Methane burns with a characteristic blue flame.

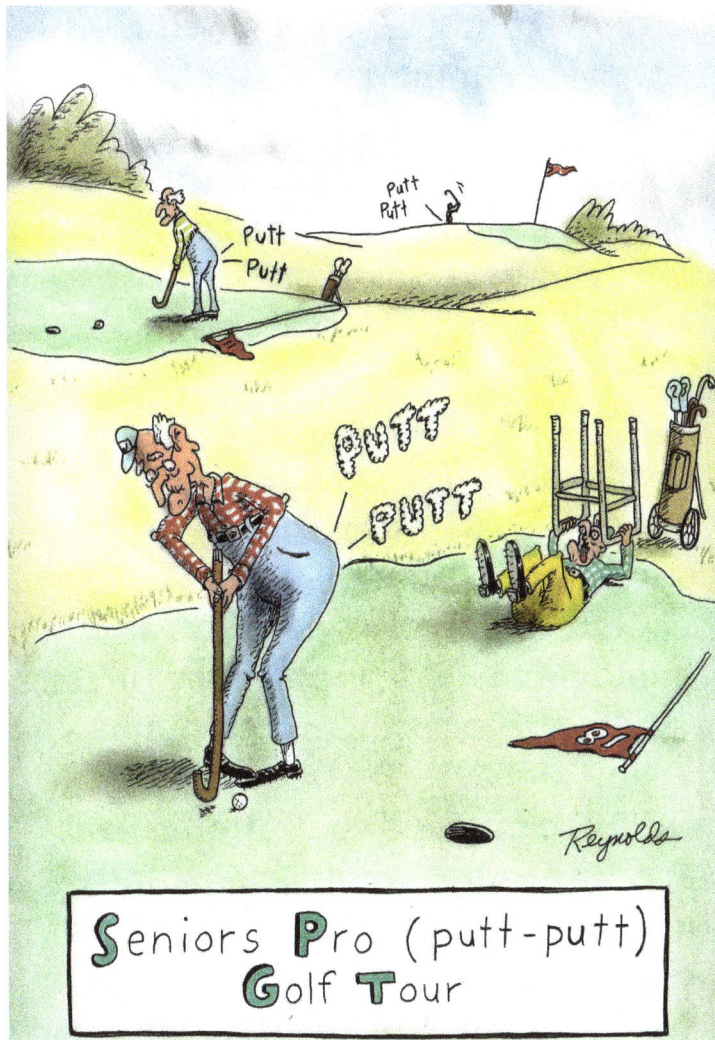

Seniors Pro (putt-putt) Golf Tour

Marcus Tullius Cicero (106 BCE – 43 BCE) was a Roman philosopher, statesman, lawyer, and orator. Cicero wrote: "The fart as well as the burp must be permitted. Cicero's *Heuristics* starts with "Open with a fart joke, use Farticus if you don't have another."

Desiderius Erasmus Roterodamus (1466 – 1536) was a Dutch Renaissance humanist, classical scholar, social critic, teacher, and theologian who was an advocate for religious toleration. His comments on farting include: "Do not move back and forth on your chair. Doing so gives the impression of constantly breaking, or trying to break, wind. Retain the wind by compressing the belly."

The Fart Side: Bottoms Up!

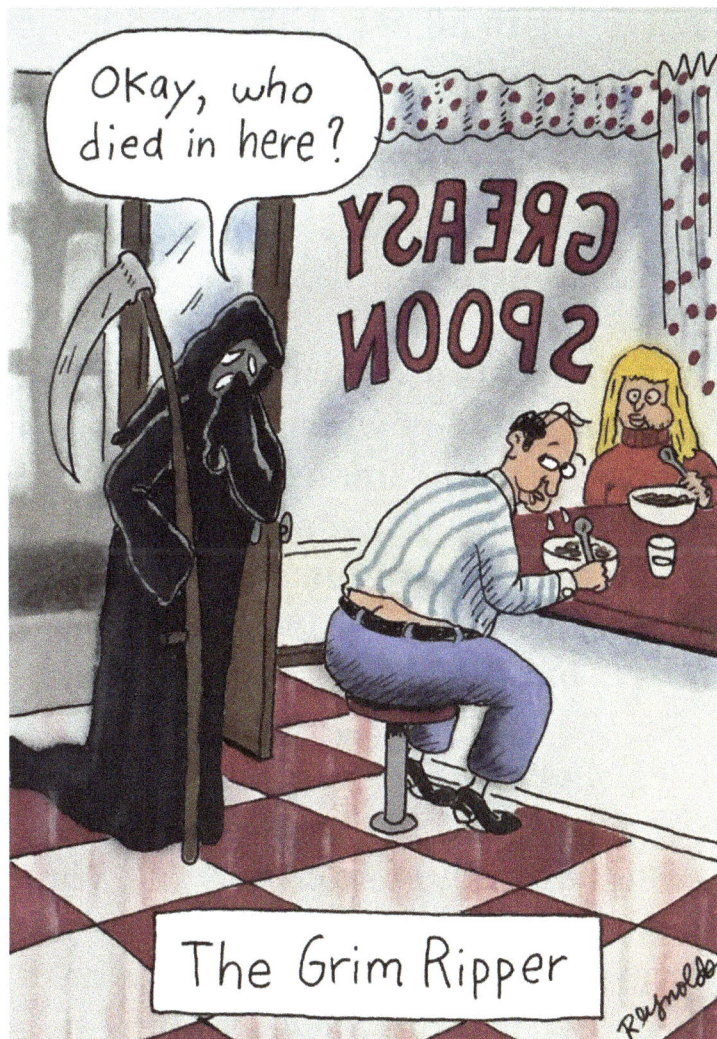

Traveling to higher altitudes, such as mountain climbing, airplane travel, hot air balloon etc. results in exposure to reduced atmospheric pressure, which causes intestinal gasses to expand.

Dogs and cats are carnivores with a protein-rich diet which produces relatively small amounts of intestinal gas, but with a pungent aroma. The dietary proteins often contain sulfur. A dog's or cat's farts are not often heard, but the odor is potent.

Large herbivorous animals such as cows, horses, and elephants, produce vast quantities of intestinal gas. The aroma is not as offensive as meat eaters because of the lack of sulfur in the protein of their vegetarian diet.

The Fart Side: Bottoms Up!

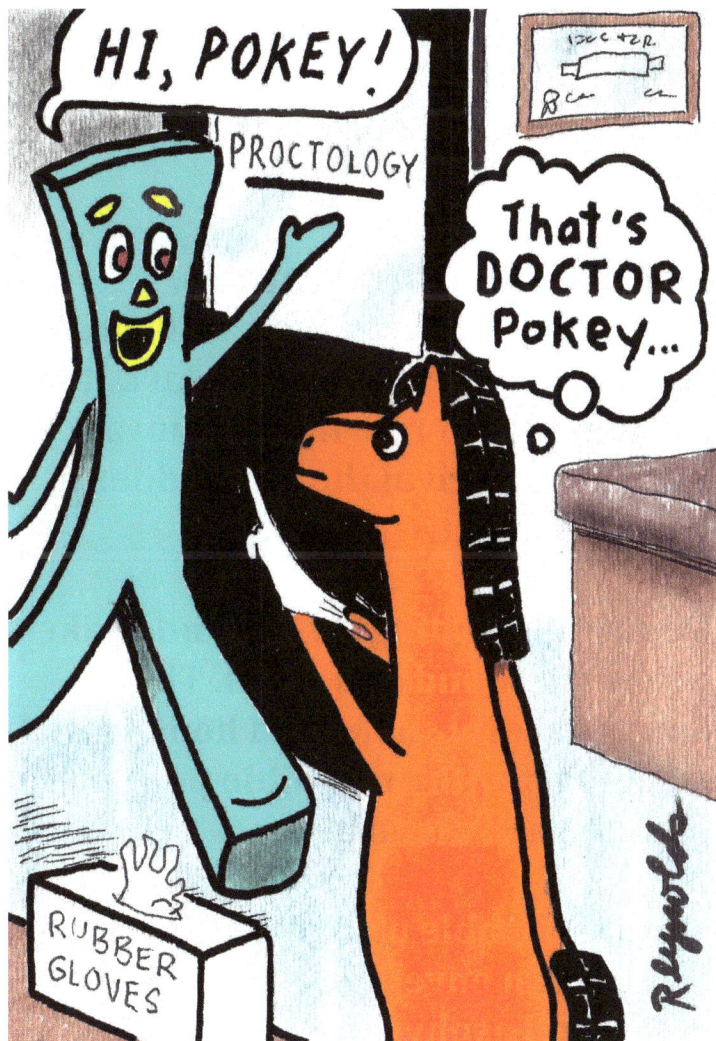

49

Fish have an air bladder, which is independent of the gastrointestinal tract, whose function is to control buoyancy.

Fish, like all living creatures, generate gas within their intestinal tract which is released as a fart. It has an unexplored role in fish buoyancy, but does not rival the air bladder in this important function.

Reptiles including turtles and snakes fart, with sound and smell. The Sonoran coral snake and hook-nosed snake fart with an audible popping sound when disturbed.

The fart bubble of a blue whale is so large it can envelope a horse and rider, and asphyxiate them both.

The Fart Side: Bottoms Up!

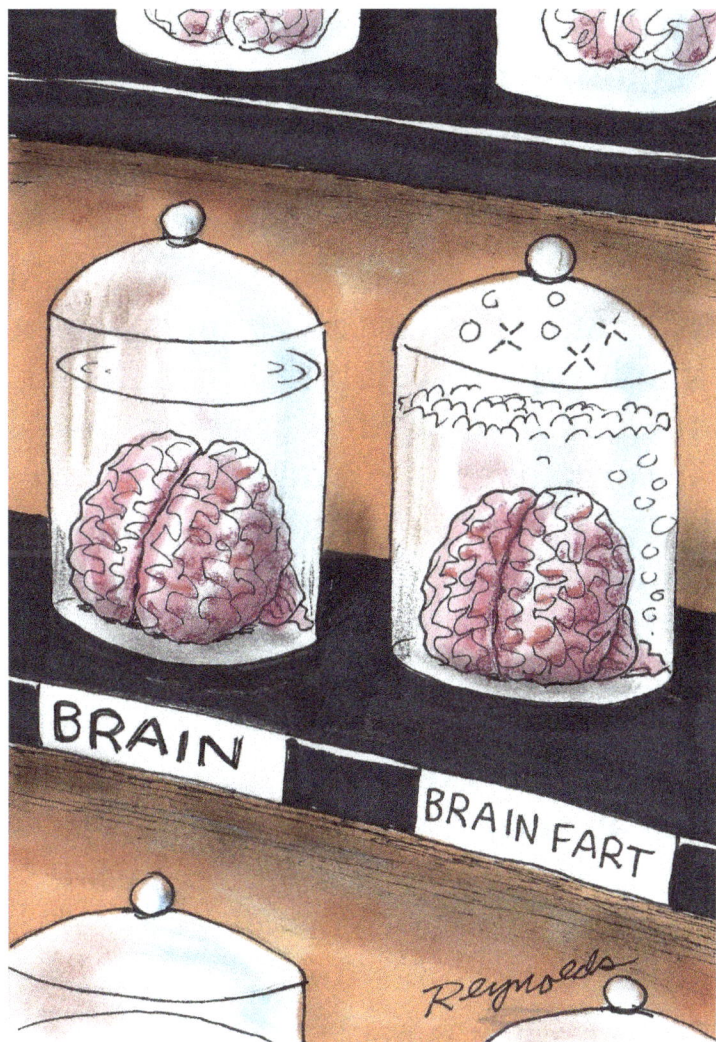

As a fart is defined as an anal escape of intestinal gas, animals that lack an intestinal or an anus do not fart. An example would be the sponge which does not have specialized organs.

The cnidarians are an animal phylum that includes the jellyfish, corals, sea anemones and hydra. Their tissues are organized into a digestive pouch with a mouth surrounded by stinging tentacles. Food enters the mouth and is digested inside the pouch, after which the leftovers are expelled via the same opening. In effect, the same opening thus serves as both a mouth and an anus. Any gas expelled by a cnidarian would be more termed a belch rather than a fart, since the animal lacks intestines as well as an anus.

The Fart Side: Bottoms Up!

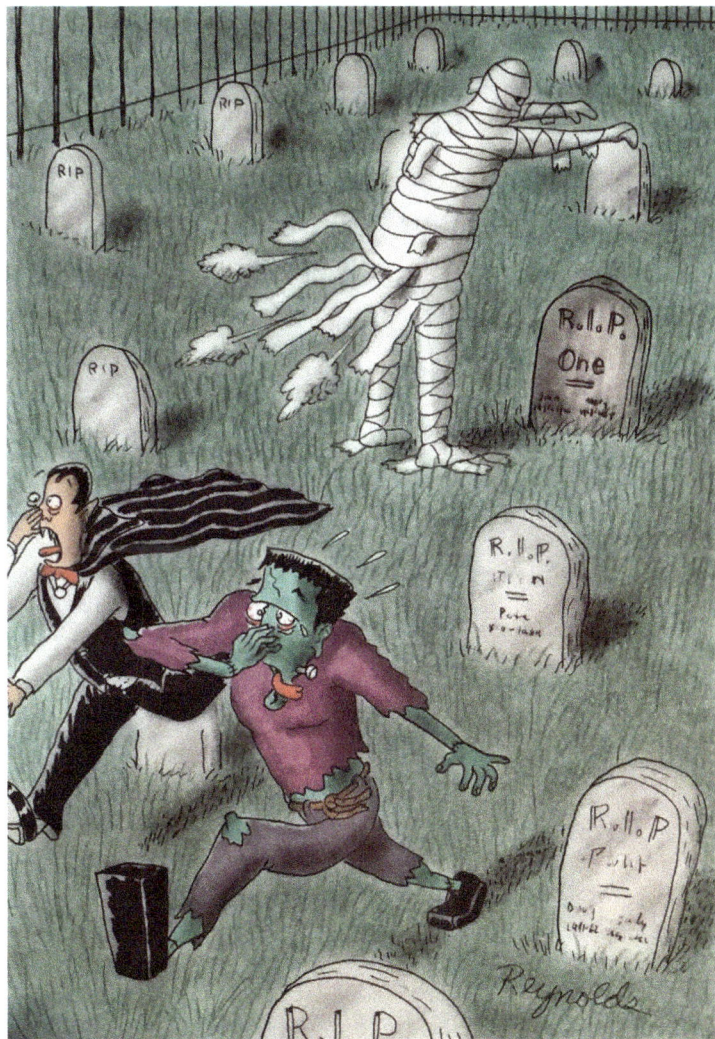

Another group of animals that don't fart are those that live very deep underwater, but nor because they do not have an anus. Living so low below the sea surface, they under enormous atmospheric pressure from the heavy volume of water above them. The pressure is so high the gas remains in solution, rather than forming bubbles. Clams, echinoderms, fish, and other animals living near the deep ocean seafloor do not fart because their gasses stay in solution and never emerge as bubbles. If they are placed in shallower waters with less atmospheric pressure, they may begin to fart for the very first time!

The explosive release of a high-pressure fart may eject a stool at high velocity, much like a cannon ball.

The Fart Side: Bottoms Up!

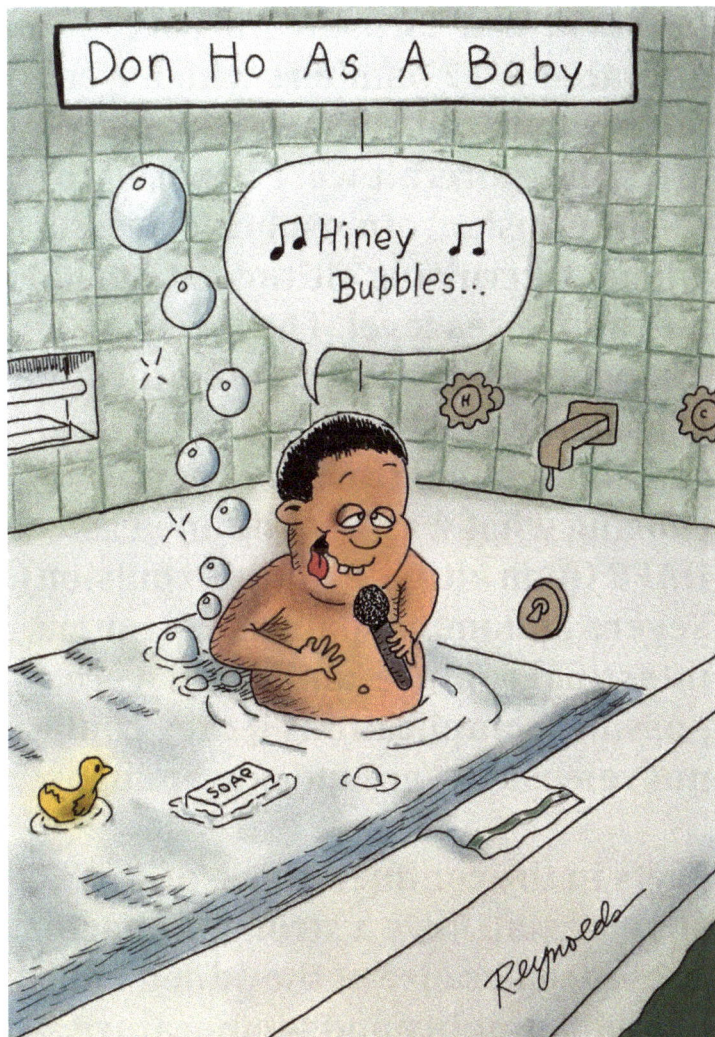

In World War Two, the Air Force operated B-17 bombers which were not pressurized. Airmen in rapidly ascending aircraft were exposed to the diminished atmospheric pressure when at a cruising altitude of 20,000 feet above sea level. The lower atmospheric pressure at this altitude caused the pockets of gas in their gastrointestinal tract to expand, causing what was later defined as HAFE (high altitude flatus expulsion). Severe abdominal pain, barotrauma, intestinal rupture, and death were possible complications if they could not release the gas quickly enough.

Farts in the confined space of a shower stall have a stronger olfactory presence because of the added effects of high humidity and temperature.

The Fart Side: Bottoms Up!

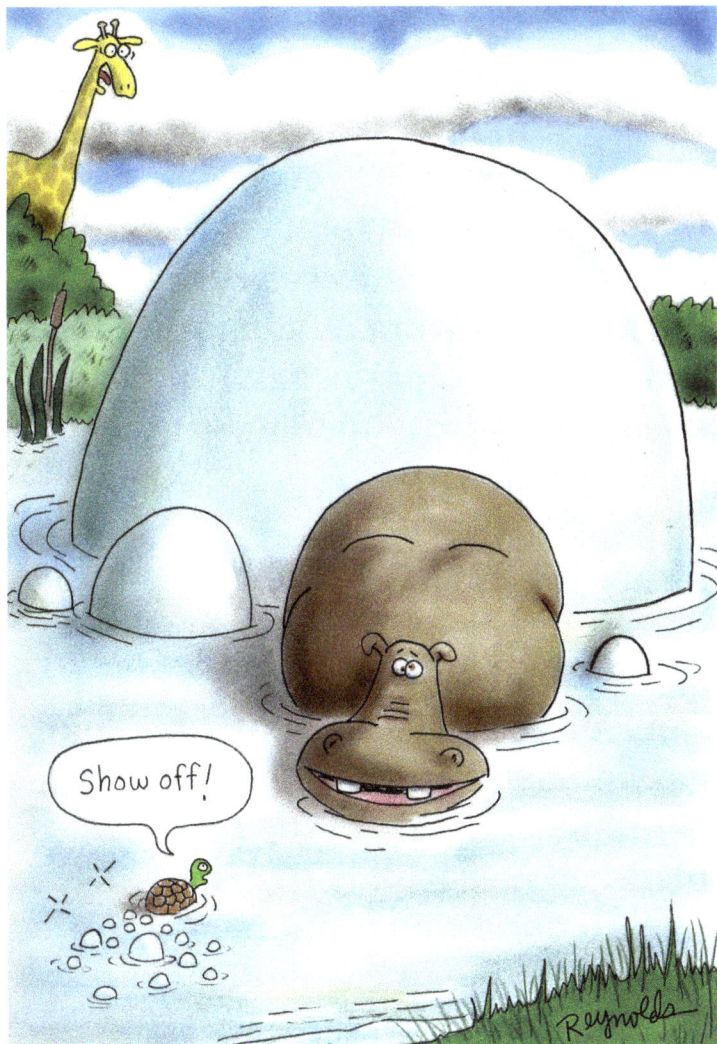

The chemical capsaicin, found in hot chili peppers and other hot spices, causes stimulation of the sensitive temperature nerve receptors. Capsaicin applied to the skin or mucous membranes results in a burning sensation. When ingested, it can pass through the gastrointestinal tract and cause a burning sensation in the rectum and anus.

A rare condition of a colovaginal fistula, an abnormal passageway between the bowel and the vagina, can lead to the passage of intestinal gas and feces out through the female genitalia. A fistula to the urinary bladder can result in urinary tract infections as well as peumaturia, air bubbles in the urine of men or women.

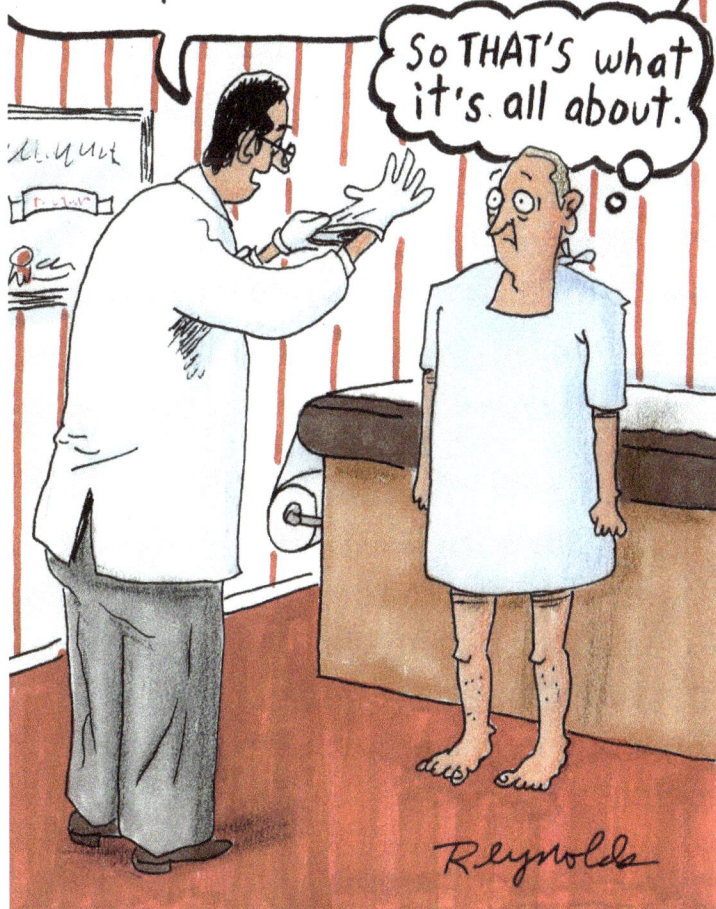

Ice cream is often forty percent air by volume, and leads to intestinal gas.

Sternutation is the formal term for a sneeze.

Trapped air in the vagina can be expelled with sexual intercourse or exertion. It is not a true fart, and does not have the characteristic odor of a fart, but it can sound like one. It is often referred to as a queef. In Great Britain, this phenomenon is called a "fanny fart." In the United States "fanny" refers to the buttocks, in Great Britain, the word fanny pertains to the female genitalia. Eructation is the formal term for a belch or burp.

Tussis is the formal term for a cough.

The Fart Side: Bottoms Up!

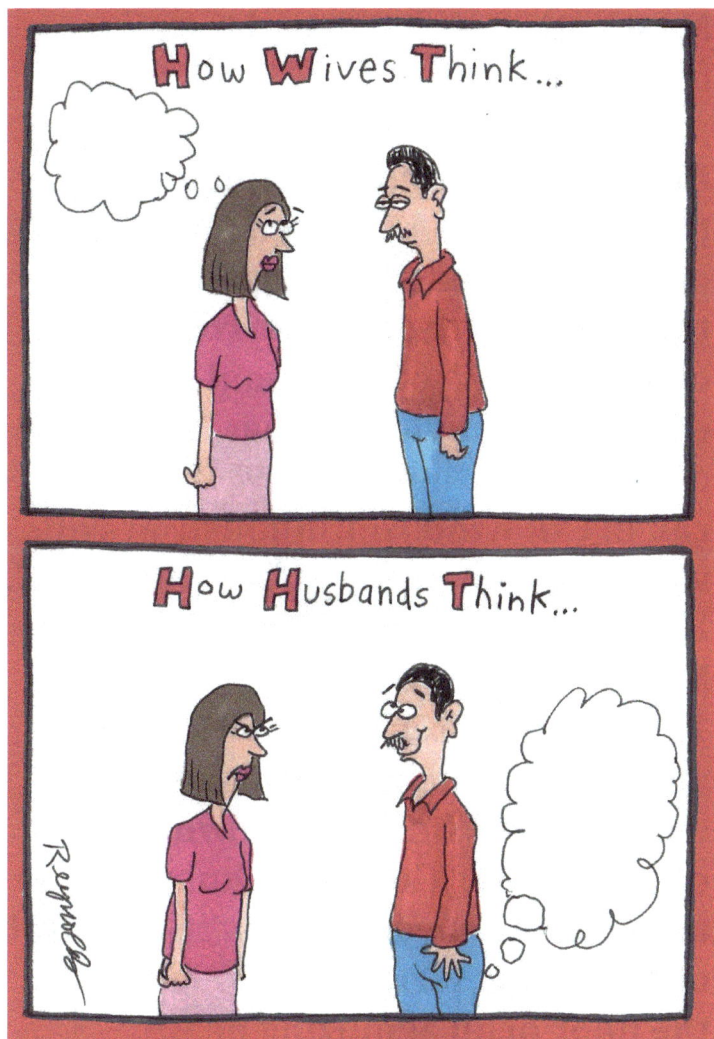

Mastication is the formal term for chewing.

Augustine of Hippo (St. Augustine) (354 AD – 430-AD) was a Christian philosopher and theologian. In his treatise on *City of God* he comments on the passing of intestinal gas. He describes individuals that "have such command of their bowels, that they can break wind continuously at will, so as to produce the effect of singing".

Michel Eyquem de Montaigne (1533-1592) was a French Renaissance author, statesman, physician, essayist, and sufferer of chronic constipation. "God alone knows how many times our bellies, by the refusal of one single fart, have brought us to the door of an agonizing death."

The Fart Side: Bottoms Up!

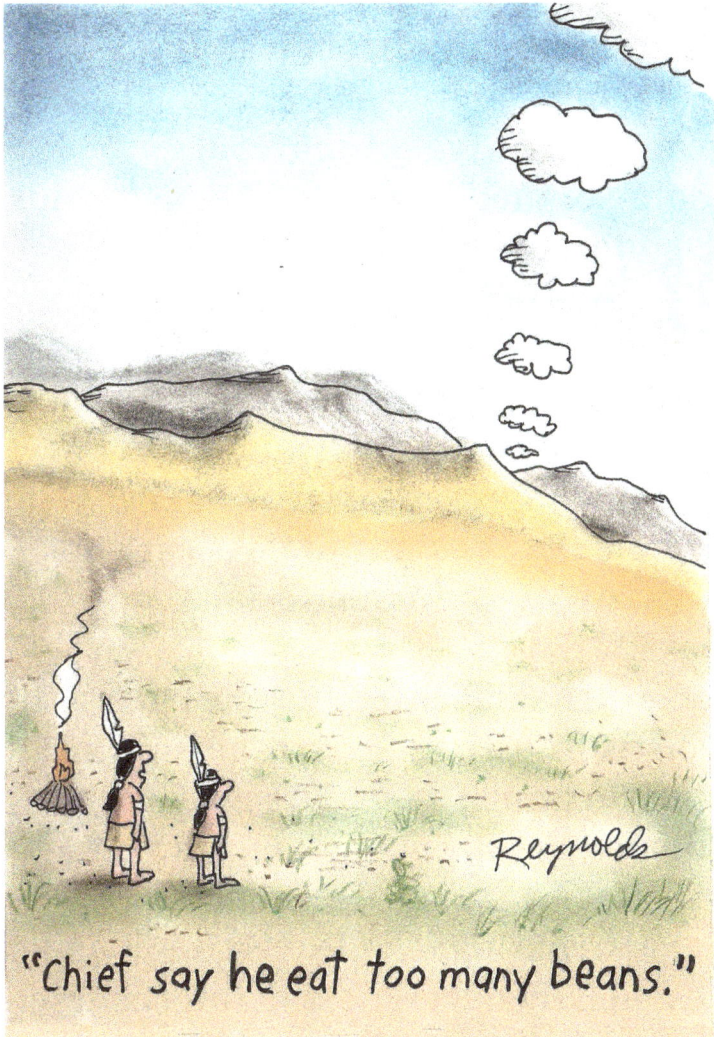

"Chief say he eat too many beans."

Farts that pass-through clothing and filtering material, especially if it contains activated charcoal, lose some of their potency. The molecules of odorants, as well as microscopic droplets of feces, become trapped in the clothing fibers. The streaks and marks on underwear are partly due to lack of total anal hygiene after a bowel movement, as well as the particulate residue of farts carrying microscopic fecal material.

If internal bleeding is occurring in the gastrointestinal tract, especially in the rectum or anus, it is possible to disperse a spray of blood with a vigorous fart. It can also occur in a menstruating female who has a queef, especially during sexual intercourse.

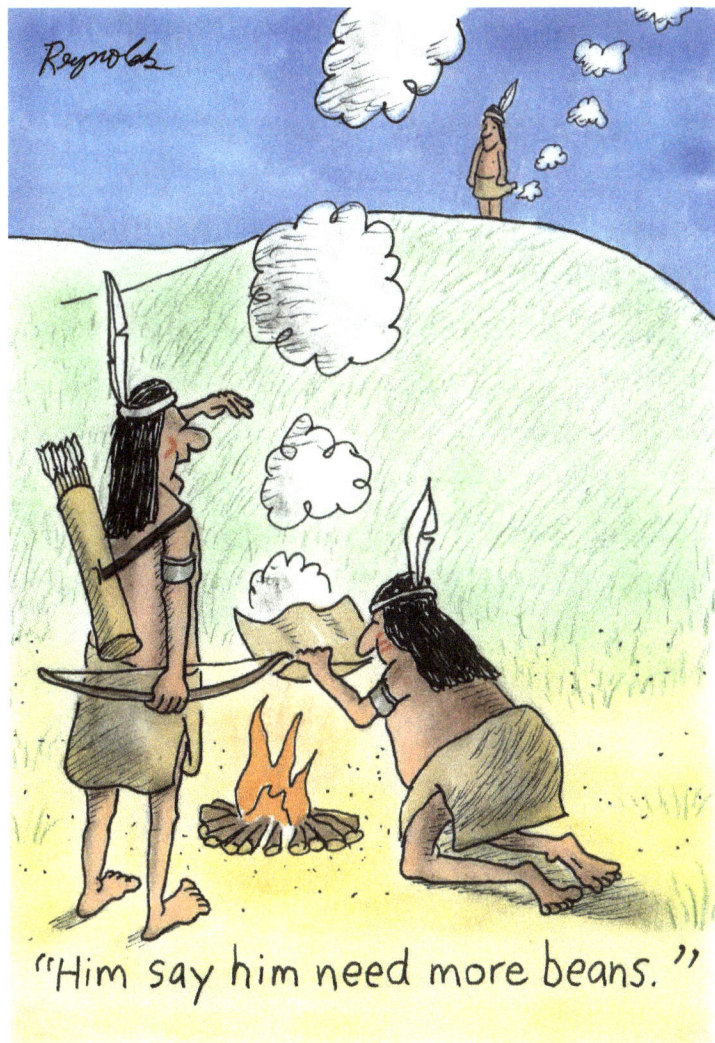

"Him say him need more beans."

When one passes a quiet fart, especially a very odiferous type known as a silent but deadly (SBD) fart, the natural inclination is to walk some distance away so as not be identified as the source. This is often a failed maneuver because the contributor's clothing retains a lingering trace, and the walking away creates a flow of turbulence of the aroma. This creates an olfactory trail leading directly to the culprit.

A space suit contains the propulsive force of a fart. Without a spacesuit, its energy would lead the body of the farting astronaut to move in the opposite direction. Its propulsive motion would be heightened because it is unopposed because of the lack of friction in the vacuum of outer space.

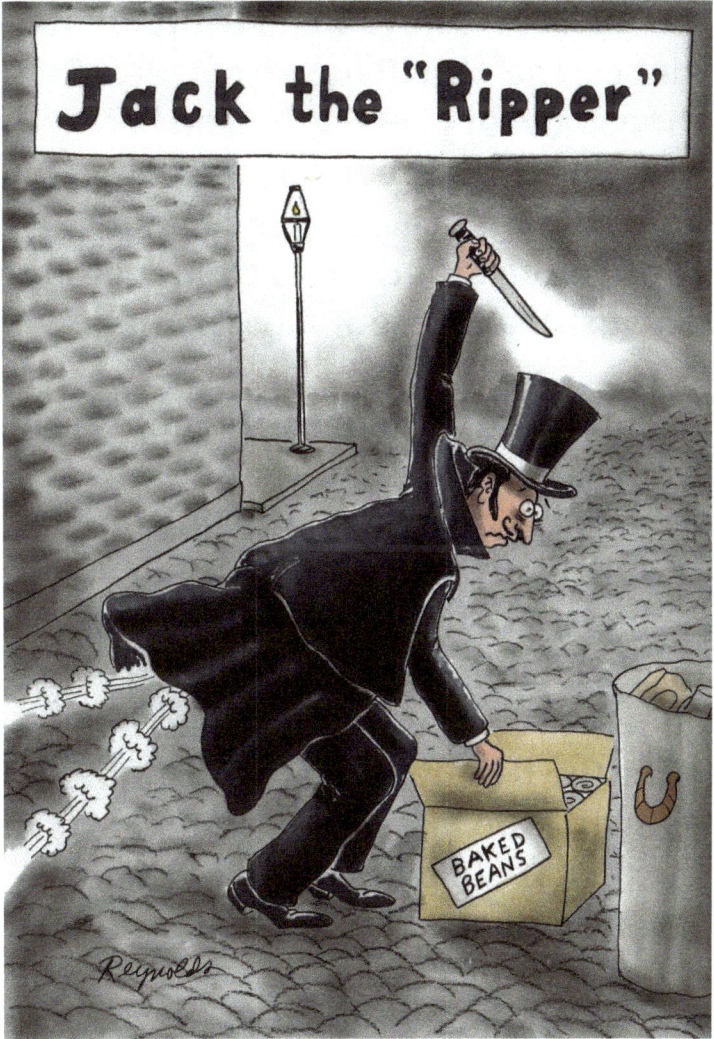

Termite farts have been trapped in amber, the petrified sap of trees, for thousands of years. Fossil farts preserved in amber have been analyzed by gas chromatography, confirming that they contain methane gas just like present day termites.

Technically, it is not the termites that generate the methane gas but the Archaea microbes that reside in the termite's digestive tract. Archaea ferment the cellulose in the termite diet. The microbes continued to generate the gasses for some time after the termite died in the amber, allowing the last post-mortem farts of the termite to be trapped as bubbles visible and ready to be analyzed thousands of years later, as their last gift to human knowledge.

The Fart Side: Bottoms Up!

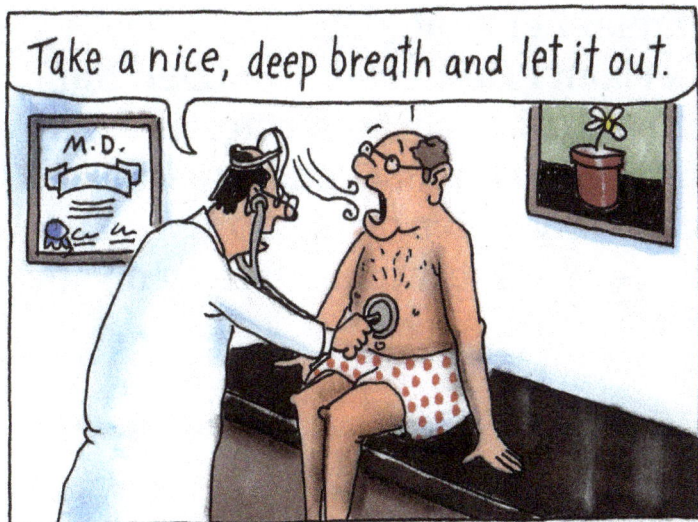

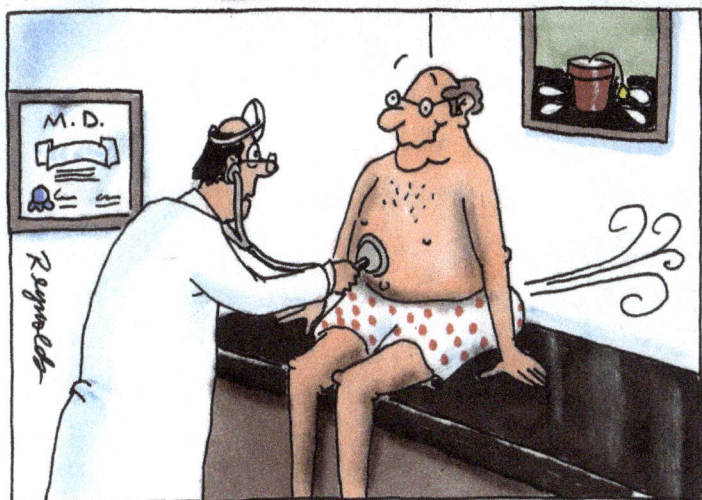

Immanuel Kant (1724 –1804) was a German Prussian philosopher. Kant described hypochondriac winds as farts when raging in the guts, and as heavenly visions when raging in the mind. Kant saw in the farting mystic a parody of himself.

Carbon dioxide gas is heavier than air.

Sir Winston Spencer Churchill (1874-1965) was a British statesmen and Prime Minister during the Second World War. At a dinner party Sir Winston reportedly farted audibly. An offended gentleman reproached him saying "How dare you pass wind in front of my wife!" Sir Winston's quick witted response was "I am sorry; I did not know it was her turn."

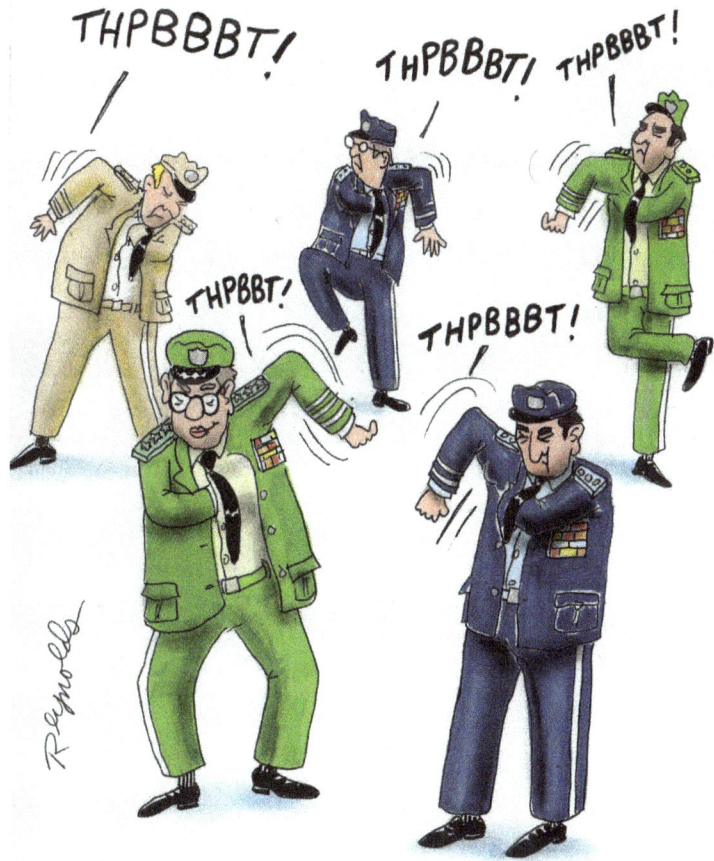

Eproctophilia is a fart fetish, the receiving of sexual pleasure and arousal from the fart of another.

Farts are found in classical art history and are illustrated by the works of Hieronymus Bosch (c. 1450 – 1516). He was a Dutch artist known for his famous triptych *The Garden of Earthly Delights*. It illustrates a nude figure farting roses, and a nude playing the flute from his rear end.

The expression "the fart of the water goblin" in Japanese means something small and insignificant. If the water goblin does it in the water, it is not heard and does not smell.

There are over one thousand six hundred known digestive enzymes.

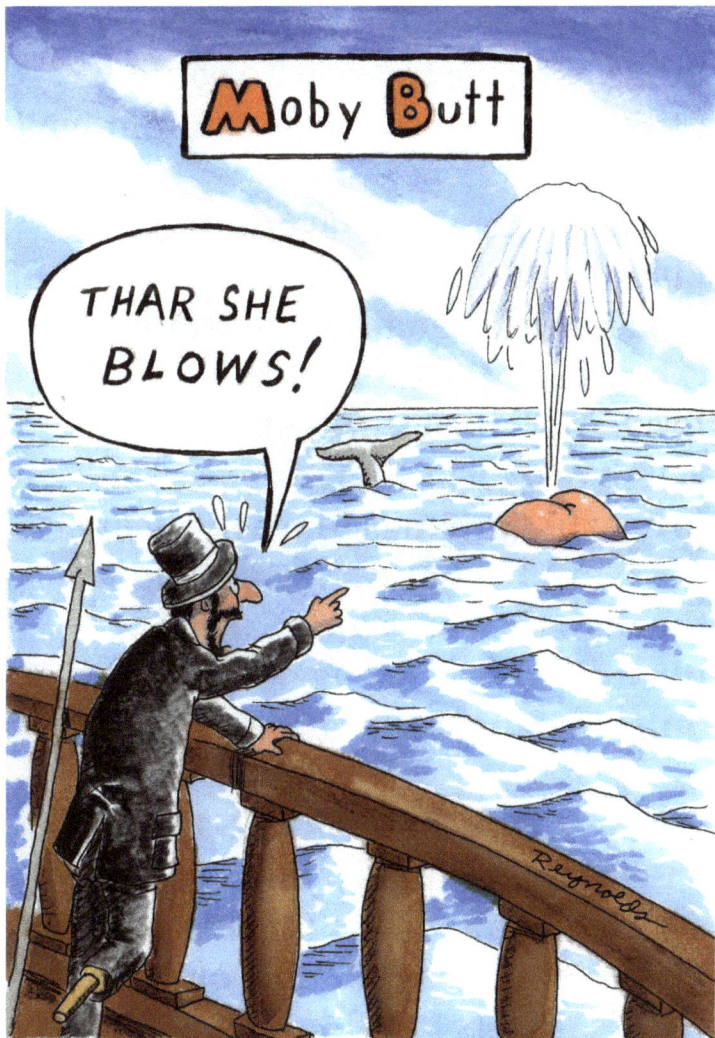

In Japan, several individuals earned a living as performers who could utilize their farts for entertainment.

Pieter Bruegel (Brueghel) the Elder (c. 1525 –1569) was an artist of the Flemish Renaissance famous for the painting *Netherlandish Proverbs* which illustrates several Dutch proverbs and sayings. The proverbs "It hangs like a privy over a ditch" and "They both crap and fart through the same hole" are illustrated by a scene of exposed buttocks above a river.

George Cruikshank (1792-1878) was a British caricaturist, illustrator and satirist. In one of his illustrations the Prince of Wales is farting on his own loyal subjects petitioning for reform.

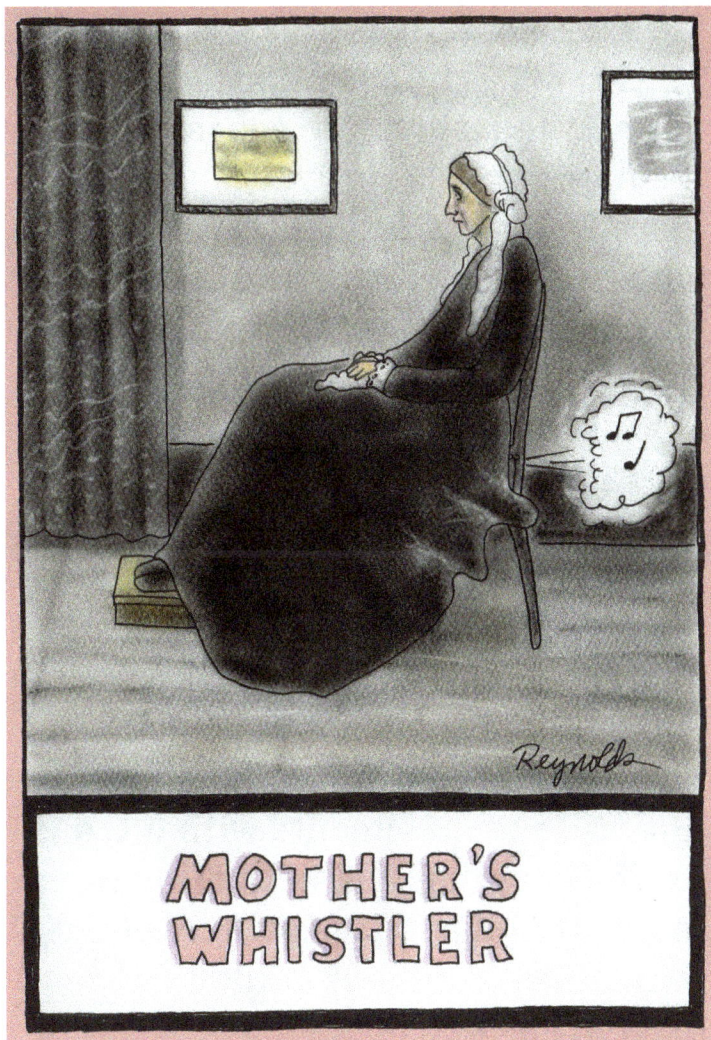

MOTHER'S WHISTLER

Wolfgang Amadeus Mozart (1756 – 1791) was a child prodigy who maintained a juvenile sense of humor throughout his relatively short but incredibly prolific and talented life. Some of his musical notes suggest the playing of a human wind instrument. He was obsessed with jokes about farts, farting, feces, analingus, and copraphilia.

James Gillray (1757-1815) was a noted English satirical cartoonist and printmaker. An etching he created entitled "Scientific Researches! — New Discoveries in PNEUMATICKS!" illustrates experiments with nitrous oxide (laughing gas) at the Royal Institution where the subject of the inhalation of nitrous oxide releases a blast of gas as a fart.

The Fart Side: Bottoms Up!

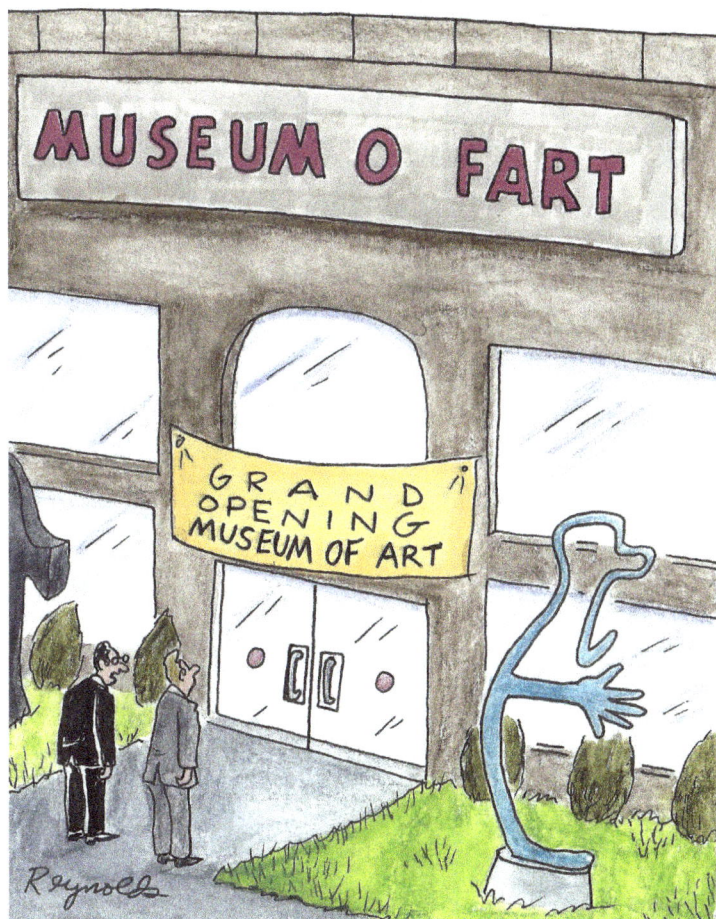

"Wait 'til the Board of Directors gets wind of this?"

Utagawa Kuniyoshi (1797 - 1861) was a great master of the popular Japanese woodblock prints and painting. Amongst his many genres he also created Japanese scroll paintings related to farting. These sell for very high prices, on the rare occasion when these prized works of art come up for auction.

Stoutshanks was a 19th century cartoonist and illustrator in England active from 1800 to 1830. He depicts the Duke of Wellington, who was then Prime Minister of England, astride a white swan propelled by farting.

Mr. Methane (Paul Oldfield) (1966-) is a British comedy stage performer who claims to be the world's only flatulist, a professional farter.

The Fart Side: Bottoms Up!

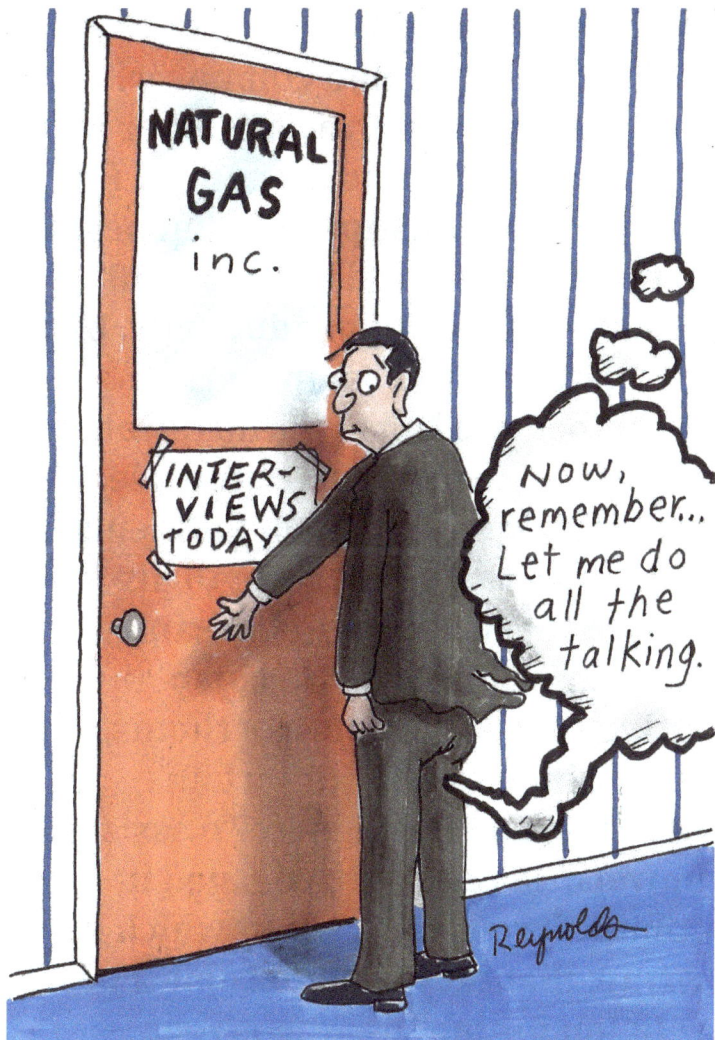

Wilhelm Richard Wagner (1813 – 1883) was a German composer, theatre director, and conductor who was best known for his operas. He had chronic constipation that began in his twenties, and he would often refer to his lack of productivity, both as a digester and composer. He described the "birth of the tetralogy out of the low E flat of flatulence." He regularly complained of flatulence in both directions, referring to his frequent eructation in the same manner as his farts. He complained in intimate details of hemorrhoids, sluggishness of his 'unterleib', bloating, and flatulence. To assist his bowels, he regularly engaged in colonic irrigations, about which he wrote, that they "had become a new religion for me".

The Fart Side: Bottoms Up!

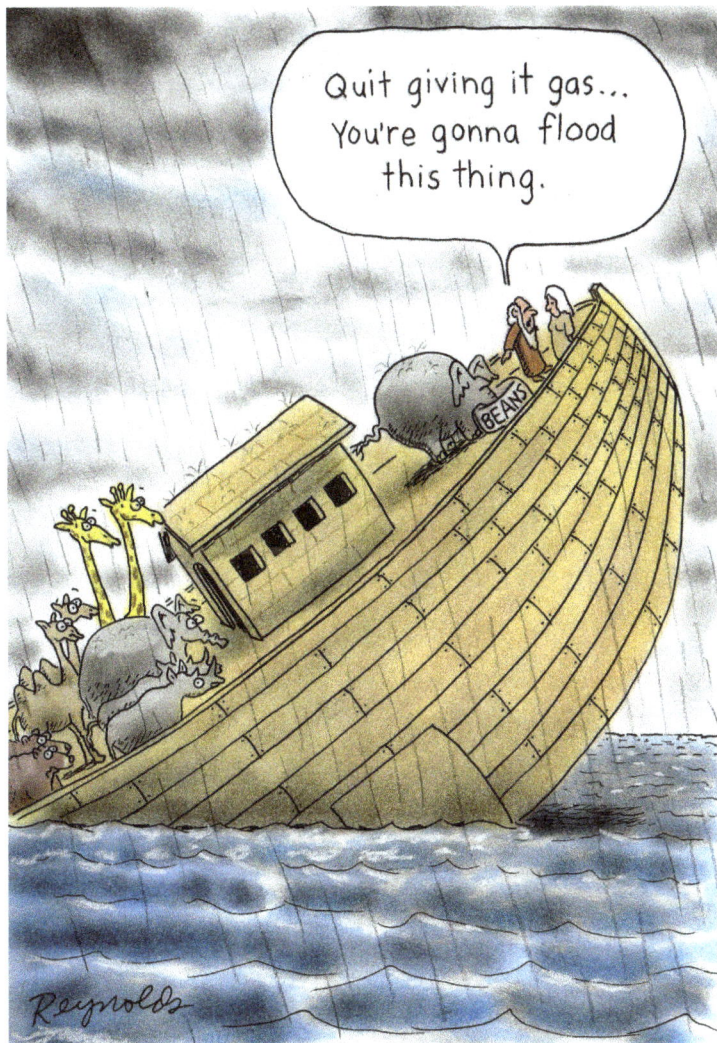

Joseph Pujol (1857 – 1945) was a stage performer from 1887 to 1914, and first performed on the Moulin Rouge stage in Paris in 1892. He had the unusual ability to inhale air into his colon through his anus, and expel it at will. With the stage name Le Pétomane, French for the fart maniac, he was also affectionately known as 'the fartiste'. He would perform musical themes on his colonic 'wind instrument'.

Salvador Domingo Felipe Jacinto Dalí i Domènechl (1904 – 1989) was an eccentric, colorful, and prominent Spanish surrealist painter born in Figueres, in the Catalonia region of Spain. He openly discussed his lifelong fascination and obsession with intestinal gas and farts.

The Fart Side: Bottoms Up!

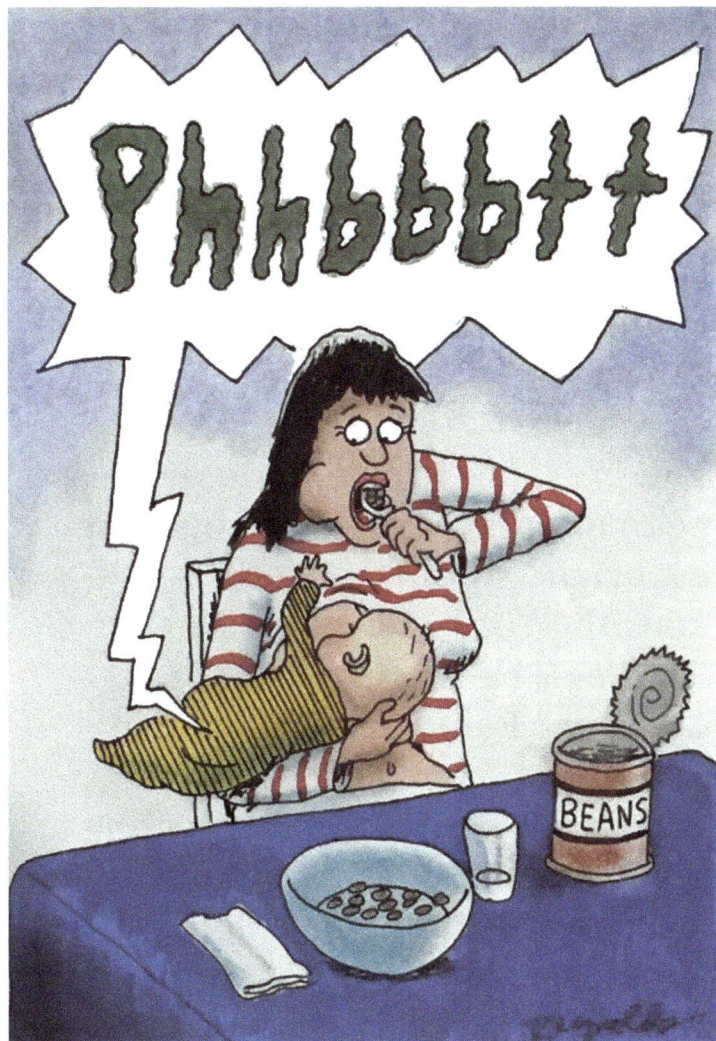

Farts have been in movies from the very beginning, you just did not know it because they were silent films. It was said that Rudolph Valentino, the suave leading man of many romantic silent films, was notorious for his extensive and pungent farting on the film stage.

The presence of cinematic farts has been out of the bag for a long time, especially since the classic fart marathon of Mel Brook's *Blazing Saddles*. The character he plays, Governor Pétomane is named in honor of the famous Frenchman, Joseph Pujol, who brought farting to the heights of the entertainment world on Paris' famous Moulin Rouge under his stage name of Le Pétomane (French for the 'fart maniac').

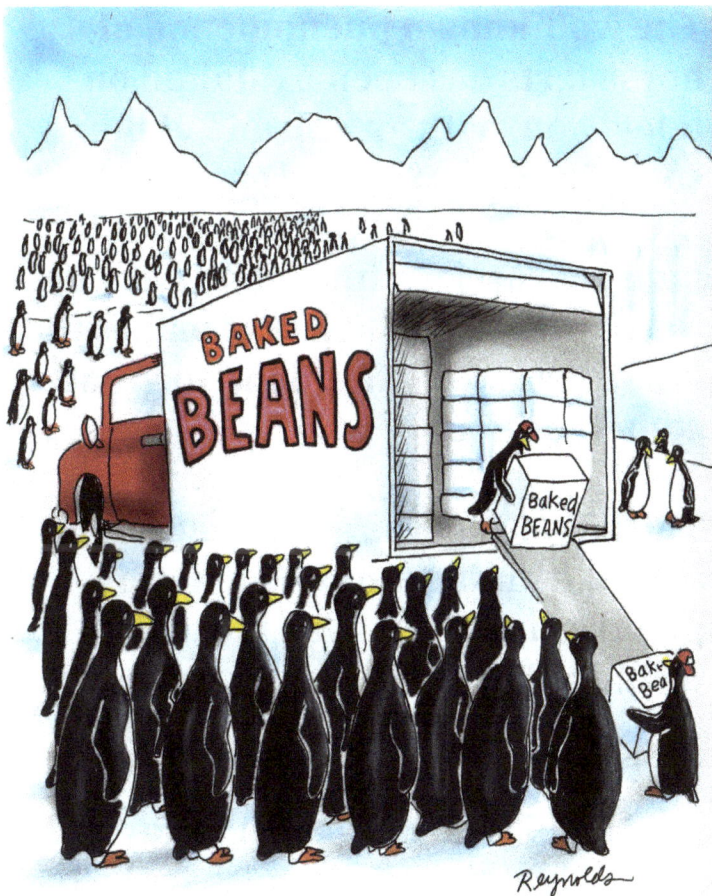

The real reason behind global warming

The well-known phenomenon of horse farts has been exploited on television, with an episode of the comedy series *Seinfeld* entitled *The Rye*. Cramer feeds the horse pulling a hansom carriage in Central Park in New York City a meal that makes the horse extremely flatulent, to great comedic effect

The Lion King was a very successful award winning animated motion picture, and Broadway musical, produced by Walt Disney Studios. The song *Hakuna Matata* has the meerkat Timor leading and the warthog Pumbaa as an ever-farting sidekick. Pumbaa nearly gets the word fart into the lyrics, until warned by Timor not to say the word in front of the children.

The Fart Side: Bottoms Up!

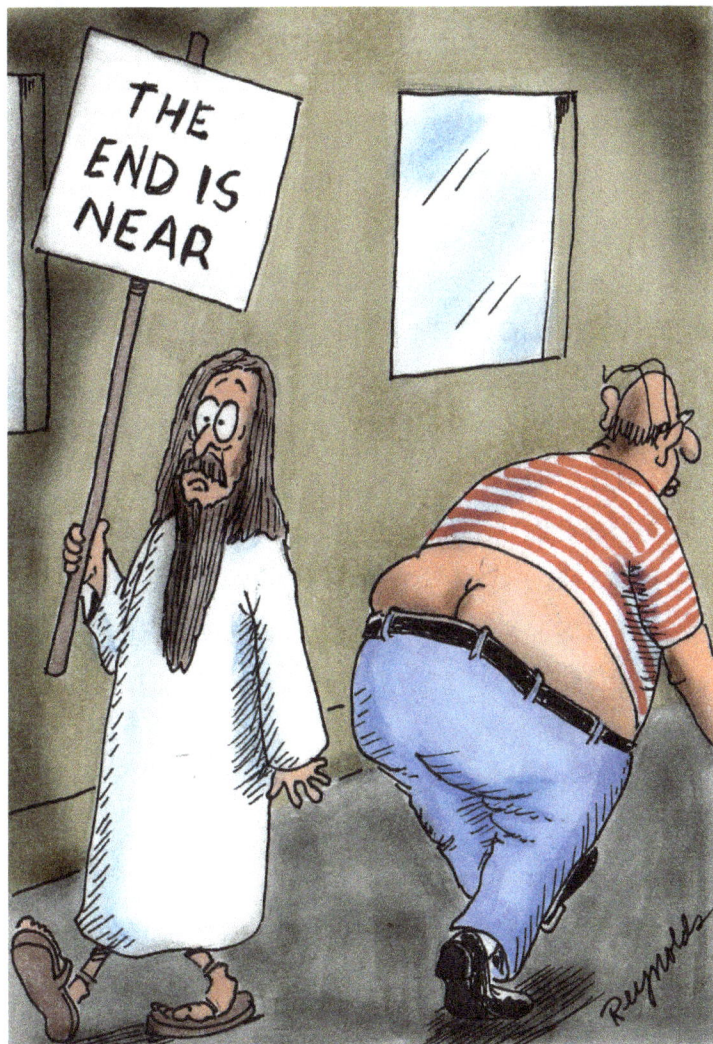

An equine fart theme took place in a Super Bowl advertisement for Budweiser beer. A man and a young woman are in a romantic horse drawn carriage. He presents her with a lit candle and reaches down to pull up some bottles of Budweiser beer. As he is bending over and out of the way getting the beer, the horse's tail lifts. The horse farts and the candle explodes in a ball of flame obscuring the young woman's facial features. When the man sits back upright, oblivious to what happened, he smells smoke and asks if she smells a barbeque.

Charles de Gaulle (1890 – 1970) French general, statesman, and gourmand, blamed his farts on dishes prepared from offal.

The Fart Side: Bottoms Up!

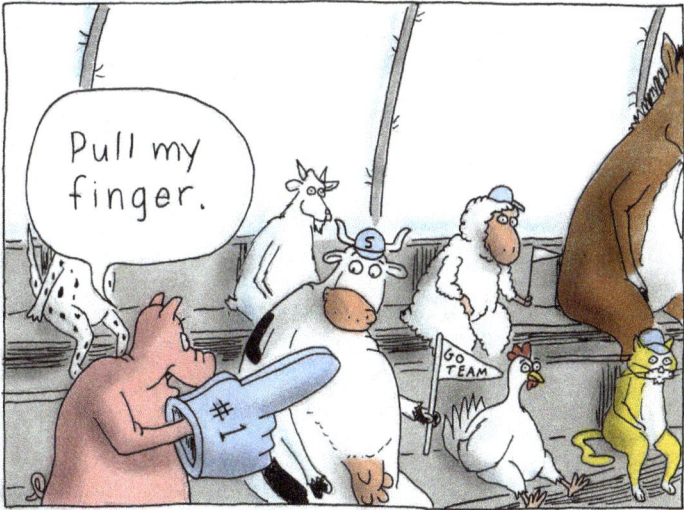

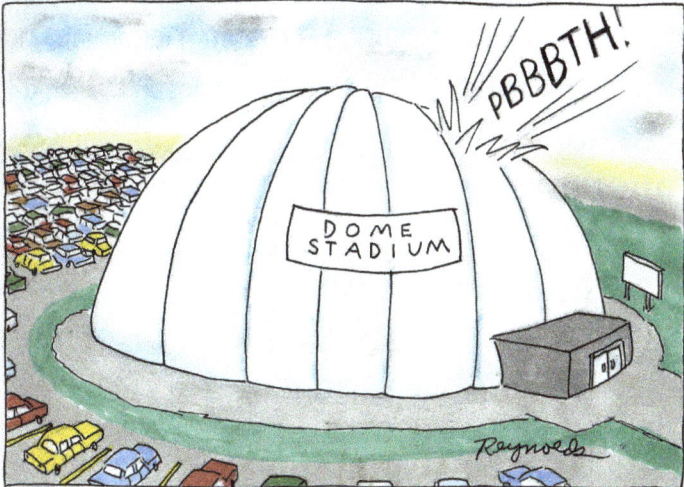

The average person swallows two thousand times per day, and each swallow includes five milliliters (one teaspoon) of air. The ten liters of air swallowed every day is seventy- eight percent nitrogen, which since it is not well absorbed, must be released as a burp or as a fart.

The musk scent gland of deer is a very expensive ingredient frequently used in perfumes. Although the word musk means testicle in the Sanskrit language it is a misnomer and is only found in the female of the species.

Toilet paper was first used in ancient China. Hardwood pulp was often used in early toilet paper and the risk of a wood splinter after wiping was a real concern.

The Fart Side: Bottoms Up!

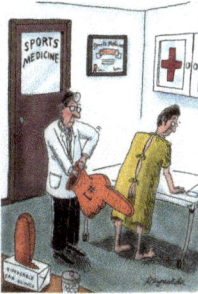
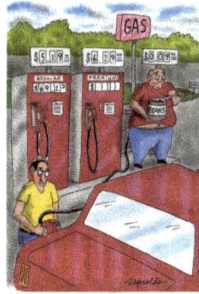
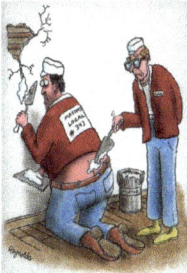
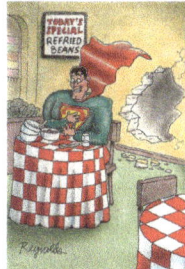

The Funny Side Collection

Dan Reynolds

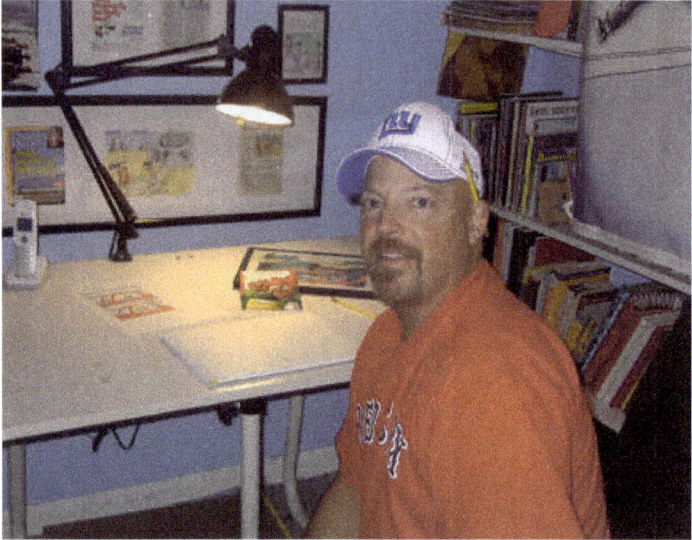

Dan Reynolds began drawing cartoons in December of 1989. He draws and eats left-handed. He plays ping pong and pool left-handed. He throws, kicks and bats right-handed. Like a box of chocolates, you never know what you're going to get, but you will like most of them and they'll keep you coming back. Unlike chocolates, REYNOLDS UNWRAPPED cartoons are not fattening.

Dan's cartoons are seen by millions of readers across the U.S., Canada, and points beyond all the way down under in Australia. His work is seen in every issue of Reader's Digest (where he is known for his cow, pig, and chicken cartoons).

The Fart Side: Bottoms Up!

His cartoons have appeared on HBO's The Sopranos, the cover of a National Lampoon cartoon book collection, and on greeting cards all throughout the United States. His work also appears in many other places as well.

Sign-up for Dan's daily REYNOLDS UNWRAPPED e-mail cartoon for only $12 for a whole year. E-mail Dan at reynoldsunwrapped@gmail.com for details. Dan's website is **www.reynoldsunwrapped.weebly.com**

The Fart Side series and other items are available at:
www.thefunnysidecollection.com

The Funny Side Collection

Joseph Weiss, M.D.

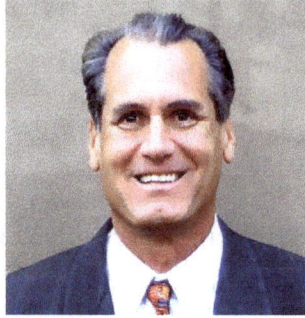

GI Joe is Clinical Professor of Medicine in the Division of Gastroenterology, Department of Medicine, at the University of California, San Diego. He is a Fellow of the American College of Physicians, Fellow of the American Gastroenterological Association, and a Senior Fellow of the American College of Gastroenterology. Dr. Weiss is the author of several dozen books on health, and is an accomplished professional speaker and humorist. His website is: **www.smartaskbooks.com**

"Dr. Joseph Weiss' books provide an informative and entertaining approach to sharing insights about our digestive system and wellbeing." Deepak Chopra, MD

"Joseph Weiss, M.D. has a gift for books that are uniquely informative and entertaining. Jack Canfield Coauthor of the Chicken Soup for the Soul® serie**s**

The Fart Side series and other items are available at:
www.thefunnysidecollection.com

The Fart Side: Bottoms Up!

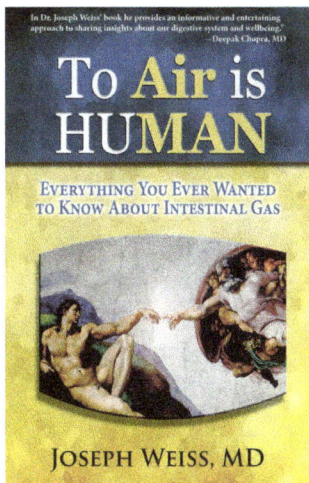

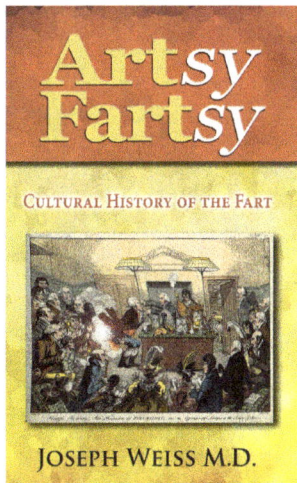

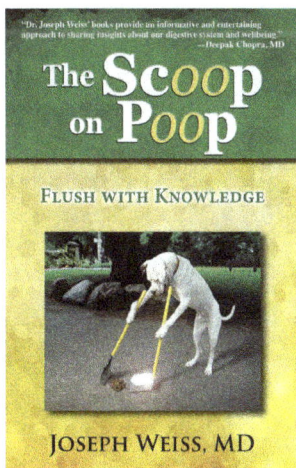

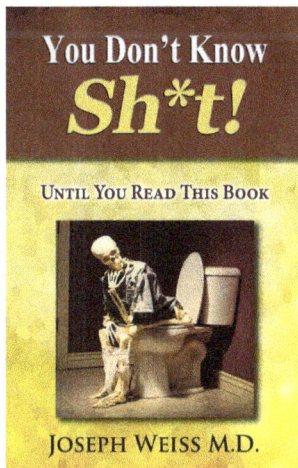

To Air is HUMAN
In Dr. Joseph Weiss' book he provides an informative and entertaining approach to sharing insights about our digestive system and wellbeing.
—Deepak Chopra, MD
EVERYTHING YOU EVER WANTED TO KNOW ABOUT INTESTINAL GAS
JOSEPH WEISS, MD

Artsy Fartsy
CULTURAL HISTORY OF THE FART
JOSEPH WEISS M.D.

The Scoop on Poop
"Dr. Joseph Weiss' books provide an informative and entertaining approach to sharing insights about our digestive system and wellbeing."
—Deepak Chopra, MD
FLUSH WITH KNOWLEDGE
JOSEPH WEISS, MD

You Don't Know Sh*t!
UNTIL YOU READ THIS BOOK
JOSEPH WEISS M.D.

www.smartaskbooks.com

The Funny Side Collection

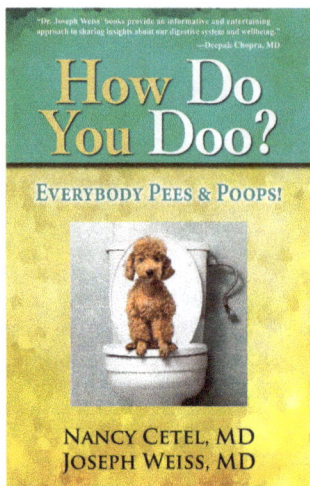

How Do You Doo?
"Dr. Joseph Weiss' books provide an informative and entertaining approach to sharing insights about our digestive system and wellbeing."
—Deepak Chopra, MD

EVERYBODY PEES & POOPS!

NANCY CETEL, MD
JOSEPH WEISS, MD

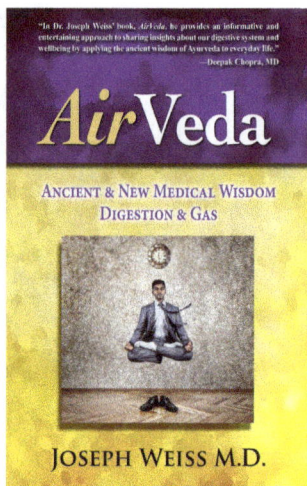

AirVeda
"In Dr. Joseph Weiss' book, AirVeda, he provides an informative and entertaining approach to sharing insights about our digestive system and wellbeing by applying the ancient wisdom of Ayurveda in everyday life."
—Deepak Chopra, MD

ANCIENT & NEW MEDICAL WISDOM DIGESTION & GAS

JOSEPH WEISS M.D.

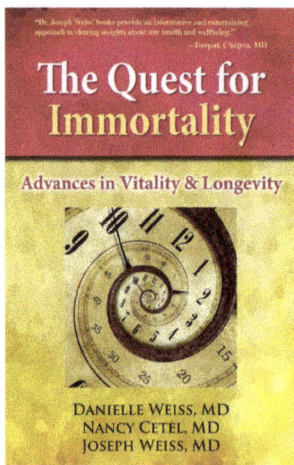

The Quest for Immortality
"Dr. Joseph Weiss' books provide an informative and entertaining approach to sharing insights about our health and wellbeing."
—Deepak Chopra, MD

Advances in Vitality & Longevity

DANIELLE WEISS, MD
NANCY CETEL, MD
JOSEPH WEISS, MD

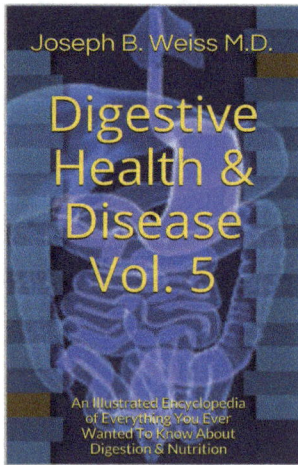

Joseph B. Weiss M.D.

Digestive Health & Disease Vol. 5

An Illustrated Encyclopedia of Everything You Ever Wanted To Know About Digestion & Nutrition

www.smartaskbooks.com

www.ingramcontent.com/pod-product-compliance
Lightning Source LLC
Chambersburg PA
CBHW071242020426
42333CB00015B/1587